100 Questions & Answers About Heart Attack and Related Cardiac Problems

Edward K. Chung, MD, FACP, FACC

JONES AND BARTLETT PUBLISHERS
Sudbury, Massachusetts
BOSTON   TORONTO   LONDON   SINGAPORE

World Headquarters
Jones and Bartlett
Publishers
40 Tall Pine Drive
Sudbury, MA 01776
info@jbpub.com
www.jbpub.com

Jones and Bartlett
Publishers Canada
2406 Nikanna Road
Mississauga, ON L5C 2W6
CANADA

Jones and Bartlett
Publishers International
Barb House, Barb Mews
London W6 7PA
UK

Chung, Edward K.
 100 questions & answers about heart attack and related cardiac
problems / Edward K. Chung.
  p. cm.
 ISBN 0-7637-1294-9
 1. Coronary heart disease-Popular works.   2. Myocardial
infarction-Popular works.   I. Title: One hundred questions and answers
about heart attack and related cardiac problems.   II. Title.
 RC685.C6A15 2003
 616.1'23-dc21

                                                    2003011836

ISBN: 0-7637-1294-9

The authors, editor, and publisher have made every effort to provide accurate information. However, they are not responsible for errors, omissions, or for any outcomes related to the use of the contents of this book and take no responsibility for the use of the products described. Treatments and side effects described in this book may not be applicable to all patients; likewise, some patients may require a dose or experience a side effect that is not described herein. The reader should confer with his or her own physician regarding specific treatments and side effects. Drugs and medical devices are discussed that may have limited availability controlled by the Food and Drug Administration (FDA) for use only in a research study or clinical trial. The drug information presented has been derived from reference sources, recently published data, and pharmaceutical tests. Research, clinical practice, and government regulations often change the accepted standard in this field. When consideration is being given to use of any drug in the clinical setting, the healthcare provider or reader is responsible for determining FDA status of the drug, reading the package insert, reviewing prescribing information for the most up-to-date recommendations on dose, precautions, and contraindications, and determining the appropriate usage for the product. This is especially important in the case of drugs that are new or seldom used. The statements of the patients quoted in this book represent their own opinions and do not necessarily reflect the views of the authors or the publisher.

Production Credits:
Acquisitions Editor: Christopher Davis
Production Editor: Elizabeth Platt
Cover Design: Philip Regan
Manufacturing Buyer: Therese Bräuer
Composition: Northeast Compositors
Printing and Binding: Malloy Lithographing
Cover Printer: Malloy Lithographing

Printed in the United States of America
07 06 05 04 03   10 9 8 7 6 5 4 3 2 1

Contents

The purpose of this book, *100 Questions & Answers About Heart Attack and Related Cardiac Problems*, is to describe for you the most commonly asked 100 questions regarding a heart attack. The book uses a commonsense approach with simple explanations so that you will be able to understand and identify easily the issues associated with heart diseases. The best way to reach that goal is through concise questions and answers.

This book describes every aspect of a heart attack, including all other medical problems that are associated with heart diseases. It includes details about coronary risk factors (factors that act to cause a heart attack), warning signs, common and uncommon symptoms, diagnostic tests, complications, and management. In addition, you can find details of various therapy methods: artificial pacemakers, cardiopulmonary resuscitation (CPR), percutaneous transluminal coronary angioplasty (PTCA), coronary bypass surgery, and implants of automatic defibrillators. As you read the questions and answers, these terms will provide you with a much clearer understanding of heart diseases and will give you the necessary tools to discuss your health with your physician.

A unique feature of this book is a summary of a candid conversation with a patient who recovered from a heart attack (Question 90). Also, the book stresses various practical and educational points as follows: What to do when a heart attack is suspected; how to prevent a heart attack; and how to live after recovering from a heart attack.

I sincerely hope that *100 Questions & Answers About Heart Attack and Related Cardiac Problems* will be a most useful, practical, and educational guide as you seek a healthy life for many years to come.

I express my sincere appreciation to my daughter-in-law, Sue H. Chung, for her valuable editorial assistance in completing this book. In addition, I express my deep appreciation to Mr. Christopher Davis, Executive Publisher, Medicine, of Jones and Bartlett Publishers, for the publication of this book. I thank Ms. Elizabeth Platt, Special Projects Editor, of Jones and Bartlett Publishers for her skillful editing of the manuscript. Last, I will always owe deep gratitude and appreciation to my late father, Dr. Il-Chun Chung, who has always provided guidance and inspiration for me.

This book is dedicated to my wife, Lisa; to my children, Linda and Christopher; to my son-in-law, James, and daughter-in-law, Sue; and to my grandchildren, Nicholas, Jacqueline, and Olivia.

Edward K. Chung, MD
Windermere, Florida

PART ONE

The Basics

What is the structure of a normal heart?

What are the normal heart functions?

What is angina pectoris or angina?

What is a heart attack?

More . . .

1. What is the usual location, shape, and weight of a normal heart?

The shape of the human heart more closely resembles a thick cone (Figures 1 and 2) rather than the more common drawing of a "Valentine" heart. The heart is situated in the chest between the right and left lungs, and it is well protected by the chest wall and rib cage (Figure 1). The normal heart size is about the size of your fist, and it weighs approximately 11 ounces (350 g) in adults. The heart can weigh as much as a pound in a highly trained athlete.

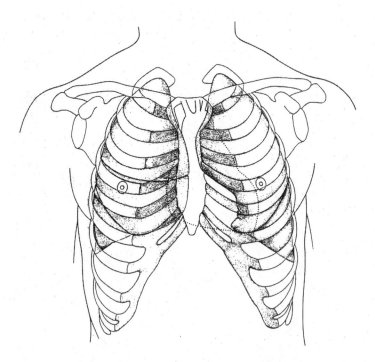

Figure 1   Location of the heart in relation to the lungs and rib cage.

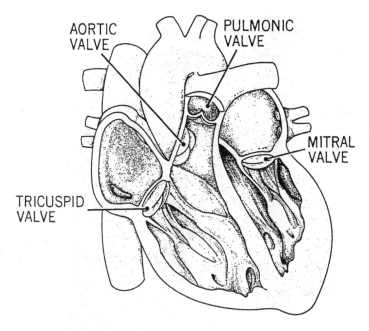

Figure 2   Anatomy of the heart.

2. What is the structure of a normal heart?

The heart is composed of muscle (called **myo-cardium**), and it is surrounded by a tough, protective membrane (or sac) known as the **pericardium**. The heart consists of four chambers; it's a muscular pump that needs a steady supply of oxygen-rich blood. The two large chambers (lower chambers) are called **ventricles,** and their main function is pumping blood. Thus, the right ventricle pumps the blood to the lungs to be loaded with oxygen, and the left ventricle pumps the oxygen-rich blood to supply oxygen and important nutrients throughout the body (Figure 3). So, the heart is not really one pump but two.

The right ventricle is situated almost in front of the left ventricle, so they're not exactly on the right and

Myocardium
heart muscle.

Pericardium
sac surrounding the heart.

Ventricle
pumping chamber of the heart.

The Basics

3

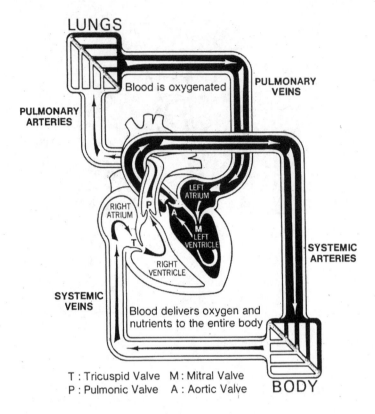

T : Tricuspid Valve   M : Mitral Valve
P : Pulmonic Valve   A : Aortic Valve

Figure 3   Blood circulation through the heart to the lungs and body.

left in the chest (if you were to look at the heart head-on). The left ventricular muscle mass is approximately 2.5 to 3 times thicker than the right ventricular muscle mass. On the other hand, the electrical energy of the left ventricle is about 10 times greater than that of the right ventricle.

Two smaller chambers (left atrium and right atrium) are located above the two ventricles. The main function of the two atria (the term atria is the plural form of **atrium**) is to receive blood from the entire body and the lungs, and the atria push the received blood down to the ventricles. Therefore, the term *pumping chambers* may be

Atrium

receiving (upper) chamber of the heart.

appropriate for describing the ventricles, while the term *receiving chambers* may be used to describe the atria.

The muscular wall between the right and left atria is called the **atrial septum**. Similarly, another muscular wall is situated between the right and left ventricles; it's called the **ventricular septum**.

3. How many heart valves are present, and how does the heart carry out blood circulation?

There are four valves in the heart (Figure 2). The **mitral valve** is situated between the left atrium and left ventricle. The **aortic valve** is located at the outlet of the left ventricle (Figure 2). These two heart valves open and close harmoniously and rhythmically to allow the blood to circulate at the left half of the heart (Figures 2 and 3). The circulation of the other half of the heart is carried out by the **tricuspid valve** and the **pulmonic** (pulmonary) **valve**. The tricuspid valve is located between the right atrium and the right ventricle, and the pulmonic valve is situated at the outlet of the right ventricle (Figure 2).

The right ventricle pumps blood to the left lung through the pulmonic arteries after the tricuspid valve closes, and the pulmonic valve opens in order to pick up oxygen (**oxygenated blood**). This process is essential for life (Figures 2 and 3). This oxygenated blood returns to the left atrium by way of the pulmonary **veins** (blood vessels that carry oxygen-poor blood and waste products back to the heart from various organs and tissues), and again the blood is pushed down to the left ventricle through the mitral valve (Figures 2 and 3).

The Basics

Atrial septum
a muscular wall between the upper heart chambers.

Ventricular septum
a muscular wall between the lower heart chambers.

Mitral valve
the heart valve located between the left atrium and left ventricle.

Aortic valve
the heart valve located at the outlet of the left ventricle.

Tricuspid valve
the heart valve located between the right atrium and the right ventricle.

Pulmonic (pulmonary) valve:
the heart valve situated at the outlet of the right ventricle.

Oxygenated blood
blood that travels outward from the lungs carrying oxygen to the rest of the body.

Vein
blood vessel that carries oxygen-poor blood and waste products back to the heart from various organs and tissues.

Aorta

the large trunk-like artery connected to the outlet of the left ventricle.

Artery

blood vessel that supplies nutrients and oxygen-rich blood from the heart to various organs and tissues.

Inferior vena cava

the large vein connected to the right atrium that collects blood from the area of the body below the heart.

Superior vena cava

the large vein connected to the right atrium that collects blood from the body area above the heart.

Cardiovascular system

the entire circulatory system, including the heart and the blood vessels.

Sinus node

natural pacemaker of the heart.

The left ventricle pumps the oxygenated blood and important nutrients after the mitral valve closes and the aortic valve opens (Figures 2 and 3). The **aorta** and its branches (which are elastic muscular tubes) then carry the blood to all parts of the body. The aorta is the largest trunk-like **artery** (a blood vessel supplying nutrients and oxygen-rich blood from the heart to various organs and tissues). It has a diameter about equal to that of a large garden hose. From the aorta, many arteries, including the coronary (heart) arteries, branch off to take fresh blood (blood loaded with oxygen and nutrients) to all parts of the body. After it delivers the oxygenated blood and nutrients to all those parts, the used blood returns to the right atrium through two large blood vessels: the **inferior vena cava** and the **superior vena cava**. The inferior vena cava collects blood from the area of the body below the heart, and the superior vena cava receives the blood from the body area above the heart (Figure 3).

Thus, the left ventricle's job is to pump oxygenated blood with nutrients throughout the entire body and to bring the used blood back to the right atrium (Figure 3). It takes about 10 to 15 seconds for the complete circulation of the **cardiovascular** system (the term for the heart and blood vessels).

4. What are the electrical events of the heart?

Electrical events begun by the heart's natural (intrinsic) built-in pacemaker (the tissue that triggers the electrical impulses) control the rhythmic and continuous blood circulation (the mechanical event). That pacemaker is called the **sinus node** (Figure 4). The

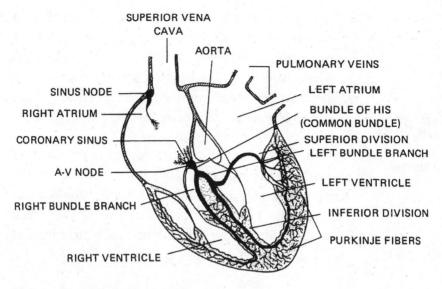

Figure 4   Conduction system of the heart.

sinus node is a small bundle of muscle fibers that contains numerous pacemaker cells, and it's located in the right atrium at the junction of the superior vena cava (Figure 4). The sinus node constantly receives signals from nerve centers in the brain and spinal cord. They respond to the demands by the body under different circumstances. In addition, hormone released by certain **glands** (in this case, the adrenal and thyroid glands) closely controls the sinus node. In simple terms, the sinus node of the heart is similar to the spark plug in an automobile. Just as the spark plug makes electric sparks to ignite the fuel and run the engine, the sinus node emits regular electrical impulses—about 60 to 100 impulses per minute in adults—to contract the heart muscle and pump blood. These impulses are what we call our heartbeat. The sinus node will continue firing these impulses for as long as a person maintains normal heart function during his or her entire life.

Gland

a tissue structure controlling a specific function of the human body, such as the thyroid gland.

The sinus node of the heart is similar to the spark plug in an automobile.

The Basics

When the sinus node fires an electrical impulse, it spreads the right atrium in a wave-like fashion from top to bottom. This electrical event is called right atrial activation and is followed by left atrial activation in a similar manner. Both right and left atrial activation produce a P wave on an **electrocardiogram** (Figure 5).

After both atria are fully activated, the heart impulses reach the atrioventricular (AV) node, another bundle of muscles located in the upper portion of the ventricular septum (Figure 4). The electrical impulse then soon passes down the "bundle of His" (the common

Electrocardiogram (ECG or EKG)

a recording of the electrical activity of the heart.

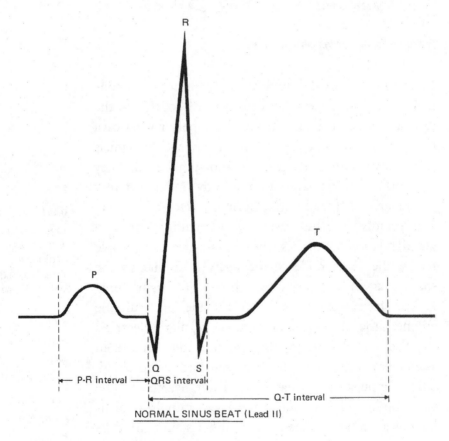

Figure 5 **Various electrocardiographic complexes.**

bundle) and right and left bundle branches in a network of His (Purkinje) fibers to set the ventricles in motion (Figure 4). This ventricular activation can actually be seen as a large wave on an electrocardiogram. It's termed the QRS complex (Figure 5), which you'll find discussed in more detail in Question 46. After ventricular activation, the ventricles relax; this stage is called ventricular repolarization. It produces what is known as a T wave on an electrocardiogram (Figure 5).

The entire electrical event started by the sinus node and ending with the ventricular repolarization stage produces the P wave, the QRS complex, and the T wave on an electrocardiogram (Figure 5). This entire electrical process makes up one cardiac (heart) cycle.

When the electrical event of the heart is disturbed in any way by various causes, various abnormal cardiac (heart) rhythms can be produced. The abnormal heart rhythm may be too fast, too slow, or irregular, or it may be no heartbeat at all. The term **cardiac arrhythmia** or cardiac dysrhythmia is used to describe various abnormal heart rhythms (see Question 57).

Cardiac arrhythmia
abnormal (slow, rapid, or irregular) heart rhythm.

A heart attack is the most common cause of various abnormal heart rhythms. Sudden death often occurs as a result of life-threatening arrhythmias, such as **ventricular fibrillation**, a very rapid, chaotic, ineffective, and irregular cardiac rhythm arising from the ventricles. You can read about such disorders in Question 57.

Ventricular fibrillation
chaotic, irregular, and ineffective heart rhythm arising from the ventricles.

The electrical events of the heart occur harmoniously and rhythmically and at the same time as the mechanical events. That is, the atrial contraction is caused by the atrial activation. It occurs immediately before the opening of the mitral and tricuspid valves. The ventricular contraction is caused by the ventricular activation, the QRS complex on the electrocardiogram mentioned earlier (Figure 5).

5. What are normal heart sounds?

During the mechanical events of the heart, the closing of various heart valves creates two distinct heart sounds. (Figure 2). You can readily hear the heart sounds through a stethoscope. When the two ventricles begin to contract, the mitral and tricuspid valves close abruptly. Then, the pulmonic and aortic valves (Figures 2 and 3) open, and the leaves of these two valves vibrate from the sudden rise of pressure caused by the blood forcing them to expand.

The heart sound created primarily by the closing mitral and tricuspid valves is called the first heart sound, and it is often expressed as "lub" if you imitated the entire heart sounds as "lub-dub." Soon after the first heart sound fades away, the pressure within the ventricles falls low enough for the aortic and pulmonic valves to close, and the mitral and tricuspid valves open.

The heart sound caused primarily by the closure of the pulmonic and aortic valves is called the second heart sound. Often, it's expressed as a "dub" if you imitated the heart sounds. Because the expansion time of the ventricle's contraction period (the **diastole**) lasts longer than the contraction period of the ventricles (the **systole**), there is a silence between each heart cycle. Consequently, the normal heart sounds can be expressed as lub-dub ... silence ... lub-dub ... silence ... and so on.

Occasionally, vibrations of the ventricular wall can be heard as the ventricles fill with blood pouring from the atria during the expansion period (diastole) of the ven-

Diastole

expansion period of the ventricles.

Systole

contraction (pumping) period of the ventricles.

tricles. This heart sound is called the third heart sound, relatively common among healthy young people.

Various heart diseases produce abnormal heart sounds in terms of timing and intensity. The abnormal noise created by a damaged or diseased heart valve is termed **heart murmur,** and various heart diseases can cause different types of heart murmurs. You can hear very loud heart murmurs even without using a stethoscope.

6. What is the pumping action of a normal heart?

A normal heart with a rate of 70 beats per minute pumps a little more than 2.5 fluid ounces of blood per stroke; that adds up to 6 quarts of blood output per minute. As a result, the heart pumps about 5,500 quarts of blood daily—weighing 6 tons! However, your heart can pump as much as 35 quarts of blood per minute when necessary, such as during vigorous physical exercise (e.g., running, competitive sports, and the like).

Your heart rate increases markedly during various physical activities. In a healthy individual with a resting heart rate of 60 to 70 beats per minute, the maximum heart rate may reach 180 to 200 beats per minute during intense physical exercise. Each heartbeat is transmitted all the way to the periphery of the blood circulation, where it is felt as a "pulse" on the wrist, neck, or ankle artery.

The system of your heart and its connected blood vessels (the cardiovascular system) is well coordinated so that it regulates the blood supply to any particular portion of your body according to what is needed there. For instance, your stomach and the rest of your digestive system require an additional blood supply during and after eating meals. When digestion of food is com-

Heart murmur
abnormal noise generated by blood flow through a damaged heart valve or a congenital heart defect.

The Basics

Your heart can pump as much as 35 quarts of blood per minute when necessary.

11

pleted, the extra blood flow to your digestive system shuts off, and extra blood supply becomes available for other parts of your body instead. During physical activity, the cardiovascular system supplies larger amounts of extra blood to your arms and legs. During any physical exertion, the amount of oxygen used by the tissues increases. For a larger oxygen supply, your heart's blood output has to be increased. This occurs primarily through a faster heart rate and more rapid breathing.

7. What is the nerve control of the heart?

Two separate nervous systems link your heart and your brain. The **sympathetic** (accelerator) system releases noradrenalin and speeds up your heart rate, whereas the **vagus** (inhibitory) system tends to slow your heart rate. The major effect of the vagus system is to depress the frequency of heart impulses fired by the sinus node.

You could compare this function with that of an automobile: the sympathetic nerve works like the accelerator, and the vagus nerve acts like the brake. Thus, your nervous system controls your heart functions according to the needs of your body.

Maintaining the normal contractile (pumping) force of your heart depends primarily upon the influence of the sympathetic nerve. This nerve increases the pumping action of the heart muscle and thus increases your heart rate.

8. What are the coronary arteries of a normal heart?

Your heart has two major (coronary) arteries: the right **coronary artery** and the left main coronary artery with many small branches (Figure 6). These coronary arter-

Sympathetic system

nerve system that speeds up the heart rate.

Vagus system

inhibitory nerve system that slows the heart rate.

Your nervous system controls your heart functions according to the needs of your body.

Coronary artery

blood vessel in the heart that supplies nutrients and oxygen-rich blood to the heart muscles.

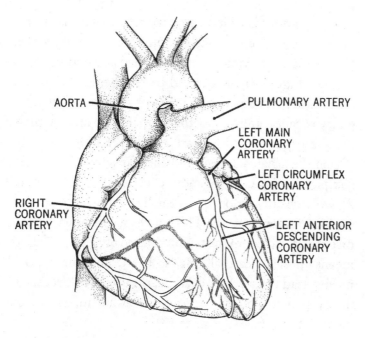

Figure 6 Normal coronary arteries.

ies, like other arteries that supply blood to other parts of your body, branch off from the aorta. Your heart has to receive oxygen and necessary nutrients constantly from these coronary arteries rather than from the blood passing through the heart chambers.

The coronary artery is relatively small, with a diameter of about 2 to 3 mm in a normal heart. In such a normal heart, the diameter (caliber) of the coronary arteries enlarges to supply larger amounts of blood to the heart muscle when the heart needs to increase its pumping action.

When the size of the coronary arteries is narrowed, usually as a result of **atherosclerosis** (hardening of the arteries), only an inadequate supply of blood to the heart muscle is possible. The narrowing (**stenosis**) of the

Atherosclerosis

hardening of the arteries, the usual cause of angina pectoris and heart attack.

Stenosis

narrowing.

13

When the atherosclerosis becomes far advanced, it may completely block one or more coronary arteries.

Coronary artery disease

heart disease due to narrowing or blockage of coronary arteries from atherosclerosis.

Myocardial infarction

heart attack.

coronary artery is called coronary artery stenosis, and it may not produce obvious symptoms in its early stage. When the narrowing of the coronary artery progresses further (Figure 7), an affected patient begins to experience chest pain, especially during physical exertion. This entity is called **angina pectoris**, or angina, often signaling the beginning of a heart attack (see Question 30). When the atherosclerosis becomes far-advanced, it may completely block one or more coronary arteries (Figure 7), which causes a portion of the heart muscle to receive no blood supply at all. This stage of **coronary artery disease** is called **myocardial infarction** (MI). "Myo" means muscle, "cardial" means heart, and "infarction" means dead tissue: thus, dead heart muscle. Heart attack in lay peoples' terms means myocardial infarction in medical terms (see Question 13).

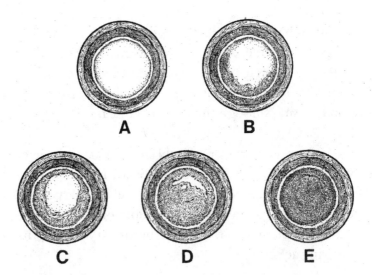

Figure 7   Various stages of coronary artery stenosis. A, normal coronary artery; B, early stage; C, advanced stage; D, far-advanced stage; E, completely occluded artery.

9. What is normal blood pressure?

A healthy heart maintains normal **blood pressure** (BP), a lot like maintaining proper water pressure in your household plumbing system or air pressure in your automobile tires. Normal blood pressure is important in keeping your blood flowing properly to your tissues. If blood pressure is too high, there's a risk of blood vessels becoming damaged, leading to the formation of plaques and blockages and, ultimately, damage to important organs like the kidneys, but if it is too low, your tissues don't get enough oxygen and nutrients to function well, causing dizziness and fatigue and, again, eventual damage to important organs. Your kidneys receive about 25% of the blood supply pumped by your heart each minute, so they play an important role in controlling BP and fluid balance in your body.

BP has two components: systolic and diastolic pressure (see Question 5). The systolic BP occurs during the systolic (contractile or pumping period) phase of the ventricles. The diastolic BP occurs during the diastolic (expanding-period) phase of the ventricles. In healthy adults, normal systolic and diastolic BP are approximately 140 and 90 mm Hg, respectively, or slightly less (see Question 24).

BP usually rises briefly during physical exercise or emotional excitement; it does not depend on the heart rate itself. By and large, BP tends to increase when you get older. The term **hypertension** is used to describe BP that is abnormally elevated. The fact that hypertension is one of the most important and common **coronary risk factors** (disorders and medical conditions that lead to heart attack) is well recognized (see Question 16).

Blood pressure (BP)
pressure within the artery during the pumping phase (systolic) or during the expansion period (diastolic) of the ventricles.

The Basics

In healthy adults, normal systolic and diastolic BP are approximately 140 and 90 mm Hg, respectively.

Hypertension
elevated blood pressure.

Coronary risk factors
various disorders and medical conditions predisposing to a heart attack.

10. What is angina pectoris or angina?

Angina or angina pectoris often is the first symptom of coronary artery disease (CAD) and, in some cases, of a heart attack. Often, angina can precede heart attack by weeks or even months prior to the attack. Angina is caused by insufficient blood supply to the heart muscle (the myocardium) as a result of one or more narrowed (stenosed) coronary arteries. It is caused by atherosclerosis (commonly called hardening of the arteries). The medical term for heart muscle damage resulting from insufficient blood supply to the tissues is **myocardial ischemia**; damage from this disorder is reversible. On the other hand, a lack of blood supply to the heart muscle caused by a blockage of one or more coronary arteries produces permanent damage to a portion of the heart muscle. Such damage is the worst event of coronary artery disease; it's what most people call a heart attack (myocardial infarction in medical terms).

Various symptoms of angina may differ considerably among individuals and can be mild, moderate, or severe. Chest pain may be a dull, heavy pressure as though a heavy object is crushing your chest. Pain may radiate to your neck, jaw, left shoulder, and arm (and, in some cases, the right arm, both arms, and the back). This pain can act as a mild burning chest discomfort, but it may also be a sharp chest pain.

In some cases, affected persons may feel little or no chest pain. Instead of chest pain, they may experience shortness of breath (**dyspnea**), marked weakness, fatigue, or palpitations (feeling of abnormally rapid heart beats). The term silent ischemia is used to describe the absence of pain in patients with known coronary artery disease.

Angina can precede heart attack by weeks or even months prior to the attack.

Myocardial ischemia

damage caused by insufficient blood supply to the heart muscle.

Dyspnea

shortness of breath.

Some affected persons may experience a higher sensitivity to heat (a warm feeling) on the skin with the onset of angina. Angina often is triggered by eating a large meal, by engaging in sudden vigorous exercise, or by feeling emotional excitement, stress, or anger.

11. How do stable angina and unstable angina differ?

Stable angina is a predictable chest pain that can be severe. Rest usually relieves such pain, and nitroglycerin (a small white tablet placed under the tongue) usually is effective in ending angina pain. Angina may occur at any time, but many affected patients experience angina in the morning between 6:00 AM and noon. The early morning hours seem to be the peak period during which most angina occurs.

Unstable angina is considered as an intermediate stage between stable angina and a heart attack, and it's much more serious than stable angina. In unstable angina, the pain pattern is unpredictable, and the intensity and frequency of chest pain can increase within a 1- to 2-month period. Neither rest nor nitroglycerin relieves the pain well. Unstable angina often occurs at rest, and it may awaken a patient during sleep. Even mild physical activities, such as walking two level blocks or climbing one flight of stairs, can easily provoke the disorder.

The early morning hours seem to be the peak period during which most angina occurs.

12. What is coronary artery spasm or Prinzmetal's angina?

Prinzmetal's angina (a variant angina) is a less common type of angina that is due to the spasm of one or more coronary arteries. Chest pain will occur almost

Prinzmetal's angina
less common type of angina due to the spasm of one or more coronary arteries.

always when you are at rest, and various abnormal heart rhythms are frequently associated with the spasm. Very often, coronary artery spasm coexists with a fixed underlying coronary artery stenosis. In severe cases, coronary artery spasm can cause a heart attack. In most cases, however, various medications are very effective in treating coronary artery spasm.

13. What is a heart attack?

A heart attack (myocardial infarction or "MI" in medical terms) is the worst event of coronary artery disease. It results from the blockage of one or more coronary arteries (Figure 8). Heart attacks are the most common cause of death in the United States and many other industrialized countries. About 1.5 million

Heart attacks are the most common cause of death in the United States and many other industrialized countries.

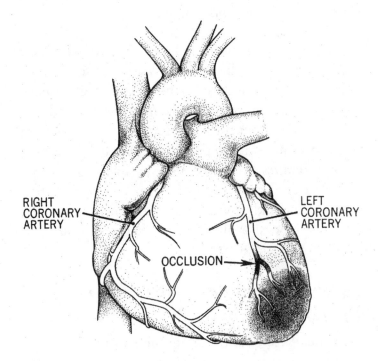

RIGHT CORONARY ARTERY

LEFT CORONARY ARTERY

OCCLUSION

Figure 8 Heart muscle showing damage from heart attack (infarcted area).

people in the United States suffer from heart attack each year, but many people recover because of advanced medical and surgical treatment. MI occurs when severe atherosclerosis blocks blood vessels, thereby interrupting the blood circulation through the coronary arteries that serve regions of the heart muscle (Figure 7). Consequently, a heart attack is manifested by dead tissue in a portion of the heart muscle (Figure 8). Recently, many medical and surgical devices and medications (discussed in Question 69 and Questions 84–86) have become available for the restoration of a partially dead heart muscle to minimize the tissue damage and to improve the outcome.

14. What causes a heart attack?

In the majority of cases, a heart attack is due to atherosclerosis of coronary arteries (explained in detail in Question 15). In the atherosclerotic process, the inner layer of the coronary arteries thickens with irregular lining, and fats, **cholesterol**, and other deposits (called **atheroma** or **plaques**) will accumulate in certain areas of those arteries. Blood clots tend to develop in advanced atherosclerosis, and such clots frequently cause marked reduction or cessation of the coronary blood circulation, which leads to a heart attack (Figures 7 and 8). In atherosclerosis, blood cells called **platelets** frequently clump at microscopic sites of injury to the inner layer of the coronary artery. This process speeds up the accumulation of the fatty deposits.

Occasionally a coronary artery spasm may cause a heart attack (see Question 12) but, in most cases, the underlying atherosclerosis coexists with such spasm. In

In the majority of cases, a heart attack is due to atherosclerosis of coronary arteries.

Cholesterol
soft, fat-like substance or lipid normally present in the body cells, tissues, and blood.

Atheroma
accumulation of fats, cholesterol, and other deposits that often lead to a heart attack. Also called **plaques**.

Platelet
a kind of blood cell that speeds up blood clot formation.

rare cases, a congenital narrowing or irregularity of the coronary artery (such as abnormal coronary arteries from birth) or a shock or trauma may cause a heart attack. Cocaine and other drugs or chemicals also may cause a heart attack in rare cases.

15. What is atherosclerosis?

Atherosclerosis (what is commonly called hardening of the arteries) is the deposit of fat and cholesterol plaques in the arteries. Atherosclerosis of the coronary arteries (coronary artery disease or CAD) is seen in angina and a heart attack, depending upon the severity of the process (see Questions 12 and 13). The atherosclerosis process begins at a young age and progresses during the aging process (Figure 7). Atherosclerosis gets rapidly worse, even among young people, if one or more coronary risk factors are present (as discussed in Question 16).

All coronary risk factors have cumulative effects.

Many disorders and conditions that we call coronary risk factors can increase your chances of developing a heart attack. Some coronary risk factors are unavoidable, but you can easily modify and even eliminate many others. It's important to emphasize that all coronary risk factors have cumulative effects, and many individuals have multiple risk factors. Typically, many obese people have high BP, elevated blood cholesterol, and diabetes, and a sedentary (inactive) lifestyle may worsen all of these conditions.

PART TWO

Risk Factors, Symptoms, and Diagnosis

Why is high blood pressure the major coronary risk factor?

What is cholesterol? What is "bad" (LDL) versus "good" (HDL) cholesterol?

How is diabetes harmful?

More ...

RISK FACTORS

16. What are the most common known coronary risk factors?

Patient comment:

When you have one or more coronary risk factors, you should try very hard to control or even eliminate these factors because their cumulative effects speed up the atherosclerotic process, leading to a heart attack even among young people. Smoking is a typical example of a major risk factor that can be eliminated entirely when you have the strong will to stop. Remember that smoking is also a very strong risk factor for lung cancer, and your family members also are hurt by your second-hand smoke.

Certain medical conditions (e.g., diabetes), disorders, personal habits (e.g., smoking), and drugs or chemicals are known to increase the risk of coronary artery disease, particularly a heart attack. Such factors that lay the groundwork for heart problems are called coronary risk factors. To prevent heart attack, you should be fully aware of various coronary risk factors. They include high BP, abnormal blood cholesterol levels, and smoking; these factors must be modified or even eliminated.

We can modify many other factors and even eliminate them altogether.

Hyperlipidemia
elevated levels of cholesterol or triglycerides (or both) in the blood.

Triglyceride
a lipid that is a lesser coronary risk factor.

Some risk factors, such as age and male gender, are beyond our control, but we can modify many other factors and even eliminate them altogether. Family history of a heart attack (the genetic or hereditary factor) is a very strong risk factor, but it can be limited to a certain degree. For instance, obesity (overweight), high BP, **hyperlipidemia** (elevated cholesterol or **triglyceride**, or both, in the blood), and cigarette smoking frequently run in the same family, but certain life styles and eating habits often influence these factors and can influence a family history of heart attack. Many individuals have been shown to have multiple risk factors. Typically, obese people have a tendency to have high BP, elevated cholesterol, and diabetes, and all that may be worsened by a sedentary life style.

Coronary risk factors can be summarized as major and minor. **Major risk factors** include:

- genetic (hereditary) factors (e.g., a family history of premature coronary artery disease);
- age and gender (e.g., men who are 45 years old and older, and women who are 55 years old and older); or women in premature menopause.

Risk factors also include:

- high BP (140/90 mm Hg or higher);
- elevated blood **lipids** (e.g., cholesterol or triglyceride or both);
- **diabetes mellitus** (explained in more detail in Question 28);
- cigarette smoking;
- obesity
- a sedentary lifestyle (being physically inactive); and
- emotional stress.

Emotional stress is a major risk factor that you might consider less important because it is not evident as a physical process. However, such stress often raises BP, and it may cause overeating or smoking from nervous tension. Anger also does not always exhibit physical signs or effects. Yet angry young men are prone to premature coronary artery disease, particularly a heart attack.

One type of minor risk factor is the excessive use of alcohol. Excessive alcohol drinking can raise BP and triglyceride blood levels, and overuse of alcohol often

Lipids

cholesterol and triglycerides.

Diabetes mellitus

the inability of the body to properly produce or respond to insulin.

triggers the onset of various abnormal heart rhythms. Nevertheless, some medical reports state that consumption of a moderate amount of alcohol (e.g., one to two glasses of wine) is said to be a protection against heart attack. Another well-known fact is that drinking large amounts of alcohol often produces heart muscle damage.

Type A personality

a person with an aggressive, ambitious, and competitive character.

Another minor risk factor is the **type-A personality**. The term type-A personality describes a person who has an aggressive, ambitious, and competitive character. Such people seem to have heart attacks more often, but this theory is somewhat controversial.

Homocysteine

chemical sometimes considered to be a coronary risk factor in abnormally high blood levels.

Homocysteine is a further minor risk factor. Abnormally high blood levels of amino acid homocysteine (a special chemical) are considered to create an increased risk for coronary artery disease and stroke. Homocysteine may harm the lining of the arteries and contribute to blood clotting. Excessive homocysteine levels are reported to occur with the deficiency of vitamins B_6, B_{12}, and folic acid, so it may be beneficial to ensure that you get sufficient amounts of these vitamins to prevent high homocysteine levels.

Endothelium

the inner layer of a blood vessel.

Other vitamins may also be beneficial in prevention of heart attacks. Vitamin E seems to reduce the risk of coronary artery disease, but its role is still controversial. Vitamin C may improve the function of the inner layer of the blood vessel (called the **endothelium**), which can affect blood flow. High intake of beta carotene and other carotenoids from dark-colored fruits and vegetables may also help reduce the risk of heart attack.

Depression has adverse biological effects on the immune system, on blood clotting, on BP, on the blood vessels, and on heart rhythms. This factor can even impair a patient's desire to comply with heart medicines. It can lead to chronic alcoholism. Somewhat related are seasonal variations: More deaths from heart disease occur in the winter months (December and January), and the fewest occur in the summertime. Short daylight hours in gloomy or rainy weather often cause emotional depression and alcoholism and therefore an increased risk of a heart attack.

Even physical characteristics can contribute as minor factors to heart attack. Some researchers have associated male-pattern baldness, hair in the ear canals, and creased earlobes with a high risk of coronary artery disease in white men.

Yet another risk factor is seen in the use of iron. A high dietary intake of iron may contribute to the process of atherosclerosis. Similarly, **C-reactive protein** (CRP) recently received special attention because CRP is shown to be one of the important coronary risk factors. Recent medical studies found the risk of developing atherosclerotic vascular disease among people with elevated CRP to be about 3 to 6 times higher than that of the general population. Atherosclerotic vascular disease, such as heart attack, is considered to be an inflammatory process of the blood vessels (including the coronary arteries). It's extremely important to measure the blood level of the CRP in the absence of any inflammatory process, particularly a cold or flu. Unfortunately, at present, no direct therapy is available to treat a high CRP blood level.

C-reactive protein (CRP)

a specific protein circulating in the blood that, at high levels, can predispose a person to a heart attack.

Some studies suggest that another minor factor—infectious agents (e.g., certain microorganisms and some viruses, such as *Helicobacter pylori*, the bacterium responsible for peptic ulcer, and the herpes virus)—may contribute to the risk of heart disease. However, bacteria alone do not cause coronary artery disease.

Until recently, estrogen was considered for many years to be beneficial among postmenopausal women in preventing coronary artery diseases, including heart attack. However, a new clinical study conducted by the National Institutes of Health demonstrated that estrogen replacement therapy no longer is shown to be beneficial in preventing coronary artery diseases in such women. Rather, this study showed estrogen to be a coronary risk factor. Further investigation will be necessary in order to clarify the somewhat controversial outcome.

Other miscellaneous factors are oral contraceptives (birth control pills) and gout. Some medical reports consider both to be minor risk factors.

Factors with potential benefits are vitamins and supplements. For example, sufficient amounts of folic acid and vitamins B_6 and B_{12} are important to prevent high levels of homocysteine. Vitamin E seems to reduce risk for coronary artery disease, but its use is still controversial. Vitamin C may improve function of the endothelium (inner layer of the blood vessel), a factor affecting blood flow. High intakes of beta-carotene and other carotenoids from dark-colored fruits and vegetables may reduce the risk of a heart attack.

17. What is cholesterol?

Cholesterol is a soft, fat-like substance normally present in body cells, tissues, and blood. It is an essential component of cell membranes and is vital to the structure and function of body cells. Cholesterol is also a building block in forming some hormones for regulating vital body functions and bile acids for digesting foods. Only a small amount of cholesterol is necessary to maintain healthy body functions.

However, abnormally high levels of cholesterol in the blood will build up on the arteries, leading to coronary artery disease, particularly a heart attack. Thus, elevated cholesterol is a major coronary risk factor. When the cholesterol level increases from 175 to 300 mg/dL, the risk of heart attack increases by almost 4 times.

Cholesterol is made in the body, mostly in the liver, and is also found in various foods from animals (e.g., meat from four-legged animals and poultry, fish, and dairy products). Egg yolk also contains lots of cholesterol. On the other hand, egg white, fruits, vegetables, and nuts and seeds contain no cholesterol.

Cholesterol has to circulate to and from the cells through the bloodstream, but cholesterol and other fats cannot be dissolved in the blood. So, cholesterol has to travel by special carriers called **lipoproteins**. Although there are several kinds of lipoproteins, the two most important are **low-density lipoprotein** (LDL) and **high-density lipoprotein** (HDL).

Lipoproteins
special carriers that are essential in circulating cholesterol in the blood.

Low-density lipoprotein (LDL)
low-density lipoprotein, often called bad cholesterol because elevated LDL is the major coronary risk factor.

High-density lipoprotein (HDL)
a cholesterol that protects the arteries against the build-up of fatty deposits.

Risk Factors, Symptoms, and Diagnosis

Normal (desirable) and abnormal (high) total blood cholesterol level ranges are as follows:

- Less than 200 mg/dL: desirable
- 200 to 239 mg/dL: borderline high
- 240 mg/dL and higher: High

Approximately 31% of American adults have borderline high cholesterol levels (200–239 mg/dL), and such people have twice the heart attack risk. The average American man consumes about 360 mg of cholesterol a day; the average woman, about 260 mg. The American Heart Association recommends limiting daily cholesterol consumption to not more than 300 mg. Depending upon the levels of total cholesterol, particularly LDL cholesterol, you should markedly reduce or even avoid the consumption of foods containing large amount of saturated fats as much as possible (see Question 20).

18. What are LDL (or bad) cholesterol and HDL (or good) cholesterol?

LDL contains about 25% protein and 45% cholesterol. LDL cholesterol causes fatty deposits to build up in the arteries. Since the LDL level affects the risk of a heart attack much more than do total cholesterol levels, medical authorities commonly use the term bad cholesterol to describe LDL cholesterol. Thus, doctors should treat high LDL cholesterol levels aggressively.

You can think of both desirable and abnormally high levels of LDL cholesterol as follows:

- Less than 130 mg/dL: desirable

- 130 to 159 mg/dL: borderline high
- 160 mg/dL or higher: high

If you have other risk factors (see Question 16) and a history of coronary artery disease, your desirable LDL cholesterol level should be below 100 mg/dL. An LDL cholesterol level of 160 mg/dL is estimated to be comparable to the total cholesterol level of 240 mg/dL. The general guidelines for desirable LDL (bad) cholesterol levels are as follows:

- 160 mg/dL or less if you have only one risk factor and no evidence of heart disease
- 130 mg/dL or less if you have two or more risk factors and no evidence of heart disease
- 100 mg/dL or less if you have proven coronary artery disease, particularly a history of heart attack.

HDL cholesterol actually protects the arteries against the buildup of fatty deposits. That's the reason for using the term good cholesterol to describe HDL cholesterol. HDL cholesterol levels in most adult men are 40 to 50 mg/dL, whereas the HDL values for women range from 50 to 60 mg/dL. The desirable level for HDL cholesterol is above 35 mg/dL. When the HDL cholesterol level is too low, losing body weight (in obese people), regular exercise, and avoiding smoking can raise it.

19. What is triglyceride?

Triglyceride is another kind of lipid. It is not as strong a coronary risk factor as cholesterol. Less than 200 mg/dL of triglyceride is desirable; 200 to 400 mg/dL is borderline high; 400 to 1,000 mg/dL is high; and above 1,000 mg/dL is very high.

You can reduce abnormally elevated triglyceride levels by losing body weight, by eating a low-saturated-fat, low-cholesterol diet, by regular exercise (see Question 23), and by avoiding smoking and excessive consumption of alcohol.

20. What are saturated and unsaturated fats?

Saturated fats are usually solid or semisolid at room temperature. They are found mostly in foods from animal origin and in some dairy products. They are also found in tropical oils, such as coconut oil and palm oil. Foods from animals containing lots of saturated fats include various meats from four-legged animals (such as beef, veal, pork, lamb), poultry fat, butter, whole milk, cheese, cream, bakery products, and ice cream. These foods contain lots of cholesterol.

On the other hand, unsaturated fats tend to be liquid at room temperature, and they mostly come from plants. These fats are usually found in common cooking oils. Whenever possible, you should substitute unsaturated fats for saturated fats to reduce cholesterol levels. You can do that best by selecting foods containing less saturated fats. Egg yolks and organ meats (e.g., liver and kidney) are particularly high in cholesterol. Sausage and bacon also contain lots of cholesterol.

Whole milk has more saturated fats and cholesterol than does low-fat or skim milk. Skim (nonfat) milk and low-fat (1%) milk have the same nutrients as 2% or whole milk but far fewer saturated fats and much less cholesterol. Butter, cream, and ice cream have even more saturated fats than does whole milk. In addition, many cheeses also contain lots of saturated fats (as much as ice cream). Thus, a healthy diet involves using skim milk or low-fat milk and eating less butter, cream, ice cream, and cheese. Low-fat cheeses, low-fat ice cream, sherbet, cottage cheese, and various butter substitutes are better choices than regular cheeses, butter, and ice cream.

One egg yolk contains approximately 213 mg of cholesterol, but egg whites contain no cholesterol. Since egg whites are good protein sources, you can use two egg whites for each egg yolk in many cooking recipes. The American Heart Association recommends eating no more than three or four egg yolks per week, including those used in cooking.

Basically, you should consume a minimum of cholesterol-rich foods (as was mentioned). If you want to eat healthy foods, you should consume more fish, skinless chicken or turkey, egg white (instead of egg yolk), low-fat or skim milk, and fruits and vegetables. Of course, proper physical exercise is also very important (see Question 23).

21. Is eating more fish a healthy way to reduce coronary risk factors? What are omega–3 fatty acids?

Patient comment:

Eating a lot of fish in place of red meat is a healthy way of reducing the risk of a heart attack. If you like raw fish, it is an excellent idea to eat sashimi or sushi at Japanese restaurants as much as possible for protein intake. Also, salmon and mackerel are good for you because these fishes contain large amounts of omega–3 fatty acids. On the other hand, shellfish like crab, shrimp, or oysters are not healthy foods for your heart.

Fish contains cholesterol, but it is very low in saturated fatty acids. Fish may be fatty or lean, but it is much better than meat from four-legged animals for reducing coronary risk factors. Fatty fish is usually found in the deeper parts of the sea and contains large amounts of **omega–3 fatty acids**. Omega–3 fatty acids are found to be protective against coronary artery disease, including heart attack.

Oily fish, such as salmon and mackerel, contain large amounts of omega–3 fatty acids. One study found that women who ate fish five times a week had a risk of deadly heart attack 45% lower than that in women who ate fish less than once a month. Another study reported that men with the highest levels of omega–3 fatty-acids had a risk of sudden cardiac death 81% lower than those with the lower levels.

Various shellfish, such as crab, oyster, lobster, shrimp, and crayfish, have more cholesterol than most other types of fish, but their total fat and saturated fatty acids are lower than those in most poultry and meat from four-legged animals. For a cholesterol-lowering diet, fish is better than lean red meat.

Omega–3 fatty acids

substances that are protective against coronary artery diseases, including heart attack.

22. What are the effects of obesity?

Patient comments:

If you think you are overweight, you should try hard to reduce your body weight because many overweight people have other risk factors, such as high blood pressure, abnormal blood cholesterol, diabetes, etc. But do it the right way, through controlling your diet and exercising—don't fall for the diet pills and other "lose weight fast!" schemes you see on TV. Get your doctor or a nutritionist involved in your weight loss. When you reduce your body weight by eating healthy foods and exercising properly, other coronary risk factors can be markedly improved or even eliminated.

By definition, obesity means 30% extra weight, and about 60% of American people are obese. Obesity is one of the major coronary risk factors. Many obese people have high BP (hypertension), elevated blood cholesterol levels, and diabetes, and they have sedentary lifestyles (see Question 23). Obesity also causes high triglyceride levels and low HDL cholesterol. Abdominal obesity (fat in the abdominal area, called central-torso obesity or the "beer belly") is a particularly strong coronary risk factor. Obese people with waist lines more than 36 inches and high triglyceride levels are at high risk for developing coronary artery disease within 5 years. In addition, obesity in children is a greater risk for future coronary artery disease than a family history of coronary artery disease alone.

23. How does exercise help in reducing CAD risk factors?

Studies have shown that coronary artery disease is nearly twice as likely to develop in physically inactive people as compared to active people. Regular moderate aerobic physical exercise (e.g., brisk walking, jogging, and swimming) for 30 minutes at least three or four times weekly will be extremely beneficial in reducing coronary risk factors.

For example, brisk walking can benefit you in several ways: It reduces the heart rate and BP, it improves blood cholesterol levels (it can actually raise HDL and reduce both LDL cholesterol and triglyceride), and it reduces your blood sugar levels. It also may open up your arteries, and, combined with a healthy diet, may improve blood-clotting factors. This type of exercise can reduce emotional stress and may promote a feeling of happiness and well-being.

Exercise can reduce emotional stress and may promote a feeling of happiness and well-being.

All individuals, however, should be evaluated by their physician to determine their ability to perform any physical exercise prior to embarking on any exercise program. That is because sudden vigorous exercise, such as shoveling snow, pushing a disabled vehicle, and mowing the lawn, are undesirable for patients with angina and for heart attack victims. Any physical activity that requires raising your arms above your head may also be risky. Other vigorous exercises (e.g., competitive sports, rapid-tempo dancing, and the like) soon after a heavy meal or after alcohol consumption can be rather hazardous. By and large, if you have recovered from a heart attack, you should avoid any competitive sport. Low to moderate physical exercise, such as walking, gardening, golfing, and moderate-tempo social dancing, is beneficial even for physically inactive people.

24. What is hypertension, and what are its effects?

More than 50 million people in America have high BP (hypertension), but more than one-half of these people don't even know it. When your BP is higher than normal, the heart has to work harder than normal. That can hasten the fatty deposit buildup that causes the narrowing or blockage of the coronary arteries. That's why high BP is considered to be one of the major coronary risk factors.

BP is expressed as two numbers in units of "mm Hg," or "millimeters of mercury," referring to the mercury that rises in the blood pressure meter as your blood pressure cuff is expanded. For example, a BP of 120/80 mm Hg is read as "one-twenty over eighty," meaning that the systolic BP is 120 mm Hg and the diastolic BP is 80 mm Hg. The systolic BP is the heart's pumping pressure, and the diastolic BP is the heart's resting pressure.

An ideal or optimal BP level is 120/80 mm Hg or lower. A level considered to be normal ranges between 120/80 and 130/90 mm Hg. High BP, the hypertension level, is 140/90 mm Hg or higher. Hypertension produces little or no symptoms at the mild level; that's why it's often called the silent killer. Nevertheless, when hypertension does produce various symptoms, they include headaches, dizziness, and nose bleeding. When BP is very high or causes major problems, serious symptoms emerge, and even death may be the final outcome. Major effects of hypertension include stroke, heart attack, **congestive heart failure** (very weak, insufficient pumping action of the heart leading to shortness of breath and leg edema; see Question 54), and kidney failure (markedly reduced functioning of the kidneys).

An ideal or optimal BP level is 120/80 mm Hg or lower.

Congestive heart failure

condition in which the heart is unable to pump blood adequately, causing various symptoms (e.g., shortness of breath, leg edema) and a common complication of severe hypertension and heart attack.

25. What are the risk (predisposing) factors of hypertension?

There are various risk factors of hypertension (see Questions 9 and 16). They include obesity, using excessive amounts of salt, lack of physical exercise, hereditary and race, and economic factors.

Obese people are at greater risk for high BP regardless of age and gender. Reducing your body weight by only 5 to 10 pounds will improve BP significantly. By and large, most people in the United States consume 5 to 6 times more salt daily than their bodies need. For some people, a high salt intake seriously intensifies high BP.

An inactive lifestyle—lack of physical exercise—can have a causal affect, resulting in high BP in certain individuals. Heredity also plays a role in high BP; it seems to run in the same family and can coexist with environmental and economic factors. Age and gender are closely related to heredity: As you age, your BP rises, and some people develop high BP. Men are at greater risk than women for high BP until the age of 55 or so.

Alcohol consumption and smoking can bring about hypertension (see Questions 16 and 19). You may not realize it, but use of oral contraceptives by some women can predispose them to high BP.

High BP is much more common in blacks and Hispanics than in whites. Socioeconomic factors also play a part in risk. People in poor socioeconomic environments exhibit a greater incidence of high BP and a higher death rate from coronary artery disease and stroke. Unhealthy nutrition with high fat and salt intake may explain these findings.

26. How should hypertension be handled?

Patient comment:

When your blood pressure is elevated, you need to have regular medical check-ups by your physician throughout your entire life. High blood pressure usually doesn't just go away, and it may require one or more medications. When your doc-

For some people, a high salt intake seriously intensifies high BP.

tor prescribes any medication, you should not stop taking it without discussing it with the doctor first. Remember that many people with high blood pressure do not have any significant symptoms, and this is the reason why it is often called a "silent killer." That's why a regular medical check-up with constant medical care for hypertension is absolutely essential.

If your BP is found to be high, you should be evaluated immediately by a physician and arrange for proper treatment. Hypertensive people must visit their physicians on a regular basis to receive proper medical care throughout their lives. Unfortunately, nearly one-half of the people with high BP are not receiving any form of medical therapy, and 30% of affected people are receiving inadequate medical care. At most, only 20% of hypertensive people receive proper medical therapy to control their BP.

The first line of management for high BP is to control or minimize all risk factors (described earlier in Question 25) as much as possible. All hypertensive people should keep their ideal body weight and reduce their intake of salt and alcohol. They should stop cigarette smoking but continue proper physical exercise (e.g., walking, jogging, swimming for 30 minutes 3 to 4 times a week). A healthy diet (e.g., low saturated fat intake) is, of course, important to reduce the risk of high BP and resulting heart attack.

When your doctor determines that one or more **antihypertensive agents** (drugs to control high BP) are called for, he or she will prescribe proper medication according to the clinical circumstance and your response. Commonly used antihypertensive medications include a **diuretic**, a **beta blocker**, **calcium blockers**, **vasodilators**, **ACE inhibitors**, and **adrenergic inhibitors**. Only

Antihypertensive agents
medications used to treat hypertension.

Diuretic
water pill that increases the flow of urine.

Beta-blocking agents
medications commonly used to treat various cardiac arrhythmias, angina pectoris, and hypertension.

Calcium blockers
medications to treat high blood pressure, cardiac arrhythmias, and coronary artery disease.

Vasodilator agents
medications used to treat severe heart failure and cardiogenic shock.

Angiotensin-converting enzyme (ACE) inhibitors
medications commonly used for a variety of cardiac disorders, such as congestive heart failure.

Adrenergic inhibitors
medications occasionally used to treat hypertension.

one of these medications can be prescribed, but often you might use two or more together, depending upon your physician's medical judgment. (Discussion regarding antihypertensive medications cannot go more fully into details because that is beyond the scope of this book.)

27. Why is cigarette smoking the major coronary risk factor?

Fifty million Americans still smoke. Cigarette smoking is one of the four major coronary risk factors (see Question 16). If you smoke a pack of cigarettes daily, you have a risk of heart attack more than twice that of non-smokers. In addition, if you smoke and have a heart attack, you are less likely to survive than a nonsmoker.

If you continue to smoke after a first heart attack, your chance of having a second heart attack increases significantly (about two to three times). Death rates increase about twofold when anyone continues to smoke after the first heart attack. Furthermore, smoking increases the risk of sudden cardiac arrest and also the chance of recurrent blockage of the coronary arteries, even after a successful **coronary angioplasty** (dilatation, or widening of the heart artery using a small **catheter**, a small plastic tube; see Question 72) or **coronary artery bypass graft** (see Question 77). Studies have shown that the chance of smokers in their thirties and forties having a heart attack is 5 times as high as that in non-smokers within the same age group.

The good news is that, if you don't yet have coronary artery disease, the risk of a heart attack starts to drop as soon as you quit smoking, regardless of how much

---

If you smoke and have a heart attack, you are less likely to survive than a nonsmoker.

Coronary angioplasty

dilatation or widening of the narrowed or blocked heart artery using a small plastic tube (catheter).

Catheter

small plastic tube.

Coronary artery bypass graft

procedure that uses a vein from elsewhere in the body, usually a leg, to make a bypass around a blocked coronary artery to reestablish blood circulation in the heart.

If you don't yet have coronary artery disease, the risk of a heart attack starts to drop as soon as you quit smoking.

or for how long you've smoked before. About 3 years after you stop smoking, your risk of death from a heart attack is almost the same as if you'd never smoked. Thus, it's very important to quit smoking before the signs and symptoms of coronary artery disease show up; if you wait to quit until after the disease is present, the risk of heart attack won't return to normal even if you quit smoking.

As the major coronary risk factor, smoking produces many harmful effects (see Question 16). Smoking damages the inner lining of the coronary arteries, allowing fatty deposits of cholesterol to collect; this impairs coronary blood circulation. Smoking increases the risk of deadly blood clot formation that leads to a heart attack or stroke. Nicotine also reduces the amount of oxygen in the blood and increases the workload of the heart by raising BP.

Smoking also negatively influences blood cholesterol levels. It elevates the blood levels both of total cholesterol and of LDL cholesterol and reduces the blood levels of HDL cholesterol. In addition, smoking often provokes a variety of arrhythmias (see Questions 57 and 58) that are very harmful or sometimes life threatening in heart attack victims or those with various coronary risk factors.

Family members who live with a smoker and inhale the secondhand smoke (often called passive or secondary smokers) also cannot avoid various harmful effects of smoking, even though the harmful effects may occur to a lesser degree. This discussion of harmful effects of smoking (e.g., predisposing factor for lung cancer) does not go into greater detail here because such aspects are beyond the scope of this book. For the purpose of this discussion, it is enough to say that a smoker or someone who lives with a smoker is at increased risk of coronary artery disease.

28. How is diabetes harmful?

Patient comment:

When you have diabetes, the most important thing you should understand is that diabetic people often do not have the usual symptoms of a heart attack. The chest pain that is the most common symptom of a heart attack in non-diabetics is often absent or minimal among diabetic people. Instead, common symptoms may be unusual weakness, shortness of breath, or dizziness. The so-called "silent heart attack" is very common among diabetic people.

Diabetes is the inability of the body (i.e., the pancreas) to produce or respond to insulin properly. If you are healthy, insulin allows your body to use glucose (sugar), but diabetes impairs this function. Adult-onset diabetes usually appears in middle-aged people, particularly those who are obese.

The risk of coronary artery disease, particularly a heart attack, increases with diabetes because the process of atherosclerosis speeds up, along with the bad influences on blood cholesterol and triglyceride levels (e.g., reduction of HDL cholesterol with elevation of triglyceride levels). Therefore, you should maintain your ideal body weight and normal or near-normal blood sugar levels with a proper diet and physical exercise. If the above-mentioned management is not effective, a physician will prescribe insulin or other medications. If you are diabetic, it's very important to be monitored by a physician to maintain proper blood sugar levels.

29. What are the harmful effects of stress?

Emotional stress can cause many harmful effects (see Question 16). Such stress is shown to be an important trigger for angina and other heart problems. Very intense stress may cause serious heart rhythm abnormalities (arrhythmias), heart attack, and even sudden death. Sudden stress increases the pumping action of the heart and the heart rate. Stress may constrict the coronary arteries and impair the blood circulation to the heart.

Very intense stress may cause serious heart rhythm abnormalities (arrhythmias), heart attack, and even sudden death.

The various heart rhythm abnormalities may become much worse, leading to life-threatening arrhythmias (see Question 38).

Stress can cause the blood to become stickier, predisposing to blood clot formation in the coronary arteries. It also can increase blood cholesterol levels, at least temporarily, and levels of homocysteine (discussed earlier in Question 16). Sudden intense stress causes high BP and can greatly increase preexisting hypertension. Repetitive stress can disturb the human immune system and may cause depression, which in turn produces a variety of undesirable effects on blood pressure, heart rhythms, and blood clotting in the coronary arteries.

SYMPTOMS

30. What are the first warning signs of a heart attack?

Patient comment:

Everyone has heard of the chest pains that signal heart attacks, but many people don't realize that the first warning signs of a heart attack may vary considerably from person to person. The warning signs may not be the usual chest discomfort or chest pain. Instead, you may experience marked shortness of breath, weakness, dizziness, numbness or tingling sensation in the arms, and even a feeling of "indigestion" with or without chest pain. When you feel these symptoms suddenly, a possibility of a heart attack should always be considered, and immediate medical attention should be sought. This is particularly true if you are an older adult with any coronary risk factor.

A heart attack usually occurs suddenly, and it can occur at any time: at work or while playing a sport, while resting or in motion. However, nearly half of all heart attack victims experience various warning signs hours, days, or even weeks in advance.

Basically, a heart attack occurs in different ways. It can be preceded by angina pectoris (angina) for days, weeks, months, or even years. Or it can be sudden, without any warning signs, and result in sudden cardiac death.

Directly before a heart attack, you may experience various signs and symptoms of angina, but these symptoms are increased for hours, days, or even weeks before the development of a heart attack (see Question 10).

The most important and common symptom is chest discomfort, including chest pain. The intensity of chest discomfort varies markedly among heart attack victims, so some people may experience little or no chest pain. The symptoms described for unstable angina (see Question 11) may worsen. You may feel a sensation of pressure or fullness, or a squeezing pain in the chest that lasts for more than a few minutes. Chest pain may spread to your shoulder, arm, and back, and even to your jaw and teeth.

Prolonged episodes of chest discomfort may accompany upper abdominal pain that differs from other

Nearly half of all heart attack victims experience various warning signs hours, days, or even weeks in advance.

forms of gastrointestinal disorders. You might also experience dyspnea (shortness of breath) after even minimal physical exertion, and this could be followed by profuse sweating, nausea, and vomiting. You would feel markedly fatigued or weak and lapse into **syncope**, or even impending death.

Most likely, you would also feel **palpitations** (due to abnormal heart rhythms; Question 57) and possibly indigestion, heartburn, and upper abdominal pain in place of chest pain. Actually, 10 to 15% (up to 30% in some medical reports) of all heart attack victims experience little or no chest pain in a silent heart attack (see Question 34).

Marked weakness can occur with or without chest pain. Among many cases of massive heart attack, the foregoing symptoms occur simultaneously. Needless to say, sudden cardiac death (usually from cardiac arrest) can occur, especially when the heart muscle damage is very large and multiple coronary arteries are blocked. A variety of **complications** (various medical problems associated with an underlying or primary disease such as congestive heart failure; Question 54) can be expected, even for those who recover from a heart attack under these circumstances.

Again, the most important and common symptoms of a heart attack are chest pain (or any other form of chest discomfort), marked dyspnea, and unusually severe fatigue or weakness. Remember that more than 15% of heart attack victims die suddenly within the first hour after the onset of the symptoms. Thus, seeking medical attention immediately is extremely important. Delay in the recognition of a heart attack and in

Syncope

loss of consciousness due to temporary cessation of respiration or circulation or very slow or rapid heart rhythm.

Palpitations

skipped heartbeats, heaviness, or rapid or irregular heartbeating as a result of various arrhythmias.

Complications

various medical problems associated with an underlying disease.

Seeking medical attention immediately is extremely important.

obtaining urgent medical treatment can trigger serious complications and even death in many cases.

31. What are the characteristic features of chest pain or other forms of chest discomfort felt by heart attack victims?

For one thing, you would feel any form of chest pain or chest discomfort deeply rather than feeling it on the surface. Physical exercise, stress, or anger often trigger chest pain, but heart attack pain does not clear up by resting or taking even three or more tablets of nitroglycerin. Heart attack victims often describe such chest pain as crushing, heavy, oppressive, or constricting, or as a sensation of severe pressure in the chest.

Chest pain frequently occurs behind the breastbone. As has been pointed out, it may spread to the left arm, left shoulder, jaw, teeth, or neck or to the center portion of the upper back. Occasionally, it may radiate to the right arm or right shoulder as numbness or a tingling sensation instead of as outright pain. Sometimes, such discomfort may be felt in much lower locations than usual, so it may be pronounced in the upper abdomen. In 10 to 15% of heart attack victims, a typical silent heart attack might not produce any pain at all (see Question 34).

32. Do women's and men's heart attack symptoms differ?

Women often experience nausea and vomiting. Pain or severe discomfort is frequently felt in the upper abdomen. Sometimes women notice only marked fatigue after everyday physical activity, rather than chest pain. Women's symptoms of angina or heart attack are not typical, so they often delay medical attention and necessary diagnostic tests.

Many women misinterpret their heart attack symptoms as other illnesses, and they have a tendency to regard their symptoms very lightly. For this reason, many physicians tend to manage this disorder less aggressively in women patients.

33. Which heart attack victims are at highest risk of death?

The outcome of a heart attack depends on the conditions that surround the event. Outcome is more serious in some people than in others. For example, elderly people (particularly those with poor general health conditions) react more intensely to heart attack. People with diabetes and diseases of other organs (e.g., kidneys, liver, lungs) also are less able to endure a heart attack. This holds true also for people recovering from cardiac arrest; those having had a massive heart attack or blockage of multiple heart arteries; and those with multiple coronary risk factors (see Question 16). People having varied complications (e.g., congestive heart failure, serious heart rhythm abnormalities, and the like; see Question 57) also suffer the results of heart attack much more severely.

34. What is a silent heart attack and whom will it strike?

The term *silent heart attack* describes an attack that produces little or no chest pain. In place of chest pain, silent heart attack makes itself known by rather uncommon symptoms: marked dyspnea (shortness of breath), extreme fatigue, and life-threatening cardiac arrhythmias (abnormal heart rhythms).

A silent heart attack may occur in 10 to 15% of heart attack cases (up to 25–30% according to some medical reports). It's relatively common among elderly people and diabetic patients. It's also more common in undereducated people and in chronic alcoholics. Such heart attacks are commonly misdiagnosed or their diagnosis is delayed because of their unusual symptoms. Thus, risk of death in a silent heart attack is higher.

35. What is cardiac arrest?

Cardiac arrest means that the heart is not able to pump the blood at all as a result of ineffective, abnormal heart rhythms: too fast, too slow, or lack of heartbeat (see Question 57). When cardiac arrest strikes, your lungs also fail to function, leading to **cardiopulmonary arrest**. (Cardio means heart, and pulmonary means lungs). Because blood circulation to the entire body, including the brain, is stopped, you become unconscious (enter a coma or a semicomatose state).

Cardiopulmonary arrest

cessation of heart and lung functions.

By and large, the underlying cause of cardiac arrest in the majority of the cases is ventricular fibrillation (as mentioned, a very rapid, irregular, chaotic, and ineffective heart rhythm arising from the ventricles; see Question 57). On the other hand, an AV block (**heart block**, slower or nonexistent conduction of the cardiac impulse from the atria to the ventricles) usually causes a very slow heart rhythm. This is a condition in which the electrical

Heart block

slower-than-usual or absent conduction of the cardiac impulse from the atria to the ventricles.

conduction of heart impulses to the ventricles is slowed or interrupted (see Question 63 and Figure 4, p. 7).

36. What are the direct causes of sudden cardiac death?

In the majority of the cases, sudden cardiac death occurs as a result of ventricular fibrillation, the chaotic heart rhythm arising from the ventricles. You can use the terms *sudden cardiac death* and *cardiac arrest* interchangeably, but the underlying problem is ventricular fibrillation.

CONDITIONS THAT MIMIC HEART ATTACKS

37. Can other ailments cause me to think I'm having a heart attack?

Many disorders, both cardiac and noncardiac, may closely mimic a heart attack. For example, the symptoms of cardiac diseases or disorders, such as **myocarditis** (inflammation of the heart muscle), **pericarditis** (inflammation of the sac surrounding the heart), and **aortic dissection** or rupture (tear of the main artery leading from the heart), can cause you to think you're going through a heart attack (see Figure 6 on p. 13).

Certain disorders or diseases of the lungs can also fool you. Some of them include **pulmonary embolism** (blood clots in the lung arteries), a **pneumothorax** (a collapsed lung), and pneumonia (infection and inflammation of the lungs). Then, too, you could be experiencing severe **asthma, pulmonary hypertension** (elevated BP in the arteries carrying blood to the lungs; see

Myocarditis
inflammation of the heart muscle.

Pericarditis
infection or inflammation of the pericardium.

Aortic dissection
a tear of main artery leading from the left ventricle.

Pulmonary embolism
blood clots in the lung arteries.

Pneumothorax
collapse of part or all of a lung as a result of accumulation of air in the chest cavity.

Asthma
recurrent sudden shortness of breath, with wheezing cough and sensation of constriction.

Pulmonary hypertension
elevated blood pressure in the arteries carrying blood to the lungs.

Pleurisy

inflammation of the membrane that lines the chest cavity and covers the lungs.

Cholecystitis

inflammation of the gallbladder causing abdominal pain.

Esophagus

feeding tube connecting the mouth and stomach.

Shingles

disorder caused by the herpes zoster virus (chicken pox) that can cause intense pain along the nerve distribution.

Anemia

a decrease in the red blood cells and/or hemoglobin content of the blood.

Vasculitis

group of disorders that causes inflammation of the blood vessels.

Figure 3 on p. 4), or **pleurisy** (inflammation of the membrane that lines the chest cavity and covers the lungs).

Gastrointestinal diseases and disorders that might fool you would be gallstone, **cholecystitis** (inflammation of the gallbladder), peptic ulcer, heartburn, and disorders of your **esophagus**. As if that isn't confusing enough, you could be having a panic attack (an anxiety attack) or Tietze's syndrome (explained in Question 43). Possibly you might have fractured a rib or be having pain in bones in that area due to other causes, such as sore muscles in the chest.

Other disorders with similar symptoms that might not be very familiar to you are **shingles**, cancer, **anemia**, and **vasculitis** (a group of disorders that inflame the blood vessels). Even exposure to high altitudes could produce discomfort resembling that of a heart attack.

Because there are so many potential reasons for your symptoms—including the possibility that you really are having a heart attack—you should not attempt to decide the cause for yourself. When such symptoms appear, go to your doctor and give him or her the opportunity to make an accurate diagnosis using the tests described in Questions 46–52. Even when it's not a heart attack, some of the other possible causes are dangerous or life-threatening conditions, so you should get treatment regardless.

38. What is pulmonary embolism?

A blood clot in one or more of the arteries in the lungs causes pulmonary embolism. Its clinical picture closely resembles that of a heart attack. However, various diagnostic tests, particularly a lung scan (a special x-ray examination) confirm the diagnosis. If you had this type of embolism, you might cough up blood.

On an ECG, the typical abnormalities brought about by pulmonary embolism (beyond the scope of this book) differ markedly from those of a heart attack. In most cases, the blood clots usually arise from your leg veins, and you would feel a very rapid heart rate. Of course, pulmonary embolism does not damage your heart muscle. This can be checked by blood enzyme tests and ECG analysis (see Question 46).

39. What is a pneumothorax?

Pneumothorax in nonmedical terms means collapse of the lungs. Pneumothorax produces a sudden and severe shortness of breath (dyspnea) that comes with significant chest pain and profuse sweating. At first glance, the clinical picture of pneumothorax mimics that of a heart attack, but x-ray pictures can point out the differences between the two disorders. Of course, no evidence can prove that pneumothorax would damage your heart muscle. Pneumothorax can occur spontaneously, for no obvious reason, but it may be caused by trauma or certain lung diseases as well.

40. What is dissection or rupture of the aorta?

Dissection of the aorta takes place in the main artery leading from the heart (Figure 6). When the inner layers of the aorta separate, thereby forcing blood flow between them, they do so suddenly, and you would feel tearing chest and back pain. Even a sharp blow to your chest could cause aortic dissection. It may happen as a

Risk Factors, Symptoms, and Diagnosis

serious complication of uncontrolled high BP. Clinically, aortic dissection effects closely resemble those of a heart attack, but various diagnostic tests can tell the difference. When aortic dissection is severe, the aorta will rupture. For many people, a dissected or ruptured aorta is fatal. However, this disorder doesn't damage your heart muscle, so if caught quickly an aortic dissection can be repaired surgically.

41. What are myocarditis and pericarditis?

Myocarditis is the inflammation of the heart muscle itself, whereas pericarditis is the inflammation of the pericardium (the sac surrounding the heart). Very often, myocarditis can coexist with pericarditis. Either disorder may be caused by a variety of viruses and bacteria, but it may be **idiopathic** (arising from an unknown cause). Nevertheless, in the majority of cases a virus is responsible, particularly for pericarditis. Often you can relieve chest pain from pericarditis by sitting up. At first glance, the symptoms mimic those of a heart attack, but physical findings along with various diagnostic tests can distinguish between the two. Affected patients often have a mild fever.

Idiopathic

arising from an unknown cause.

42. Can gastrointestinal diseases or disorders act like a heart attack?

In some instances, various gastrointestinal diseases or disorders can cause you to think you're undergoing a heart attack. Heartburn, for example, occurs when stomach (gastric) acid washes up from the stomach into the esophagus. Heartburn can produce a burning sensation behind the breastbone (sternum). Chest pain due to heartburn usually occurs after you eat a meal and may last for hours. Heartburn tends to occur more often when you bend forward at the waist or lie down. Often it's accompanied by a sour taste and the feeling of food reentering your mouth (regurgitation, a medical term for vomiting).

Other disorders that can imitate the symptoms of a heart attack center on the esophagus. They, too, cause chest pain similar to that of a heart attack. They include esophageal spasm, **esophagitis** (inflammation of the esophagus), and **achalasia** (explained below).

In esophageal spasm (spasm of the esophagus), the muscles that normally move foods down your esophagus while swallowing lose their coordination. This can lead to painful muscle spasms. Since both esophageal spasm and angina (see Question 10) can be relieved by nitroglycerin, you might mistake this condition for angina or even heart attack.

Another swallowing disorder, achalasia, causes chest pain. What happens when achlasia occurs is that the valve in your lower esophagus fails to open properly to allow food to enter your stomach. Instead, the food backs up into the esophagus (regurgitation, or vomiting), and that action produces chest pain and heartburn. Esophagitis, an inflammation of the esophagus, also can cause chest pain.

Diseases or disorders of the gallbladder, such as gallstones (stones that form in your gallbladder) and

Esophagitis
inflammation of the esophagus.

Achalasia
disorder in which the valve in the lower esophagus fails to open properly to allow food to enter the stomach. Instead, food backs up into the esophagus, leading to chest pain.

cholecystitis (inflammation of the gallbladder), produce upper abdominal pain that on the surface might cause you to think you were having a heart attack. In the majority of cases, however, the characteristic symptoms and various diagnostic tests can distinguish one from the other.

Sometimes, peptic ulcer pain may feel like that of a heart attack. If you experienced a bout of peptic ulcer, however, you probably would have a history of stomach trouble for weeks, months, or even years. The pain is always related to food.

Hiatal hernia is the bursting or splitting of a portion of your stomach into your chest through the hiatus (space or gap) between your diaphragm (a muscle that separates various intestinal organs from the chest cavity) and your esophagus. This hiatal hernia also causes chest pain that may on the surface mimic pain from angina or a heart attack. However, once again, the characteristic clinical picture and various diagnostic tests can identify which is which.

43. What is Tietze's syndrome?

Tietze's syndrome is a form of **costochondritis**. In this disorder, the cartilage (a fibrous connective tissue) of your rib cage, particularly the cartilage that joins your ribs to your sternum (breastbone), becomes inflamed from an unknown cause. The pain of Tietze's syndrome may occur suddenly, and it can be severe. Naturally, you might think you were having a heart attack, because the pain can be similar. However, this pain can always be reproduced or increased by pressure directly on your rib cage, particularly on your sternum or the ribs near your breastbone. In a heart attack, on

Hiatal hernia

herniation of a portion of the stomach through the diaphragmatic-esophageal hiatus into the chest, leading to chest pain.

Tietze's syndrome

a condition in which the cartilage of the rib cage, particularly that joining the ribs to the sternum (breastbone), becomes inflamed due to unknown causes and often triggers chest pain.

Costochondritis

inflammation of the rib cartilage.

the other hand, direct pressure on the chest wall would not influence your pain. Heart disease is not associated with Tietze's syndrome.

44. What is a panic attack?

For certain people, an unusual fear can cause an intense anxiety reaction. That can bring on chest pain, rapid heartbeats, hyperventilation (rapid breathing), profuse sweating, and shortness of breath. A panic attack may on the surface imitate a heart attack, but there is no relationship between the two. Panic attacks are a form of emotional disorder that seems to run in families, and they can be treated successfully in most cases.

45. Can bone and muscle diseases and disorders cause pain like that of a heart attack?

Injured chest muscles or ribs, particularly a broken (fractured) rib due to any number of injuries, can produce severe pain that may resemble pain from a heart attack. However, as in treating most other mimicking disorders, your doctor would be able to arrive at a diagnosis by asking you about your symptoms and by chest x-ray examination and other diagnostic tests. Sore muscles due to vigorous physical activities, particularly competitive sports, also may cause pain in the chest, shoulders, and arms. Severe arthritis of the ribs may cause pain, sometimes similar to cardiac pain.

Another disorder that can imitate the pain of a heart attack is shingles (herpes zoster in medical terms). A virus (the same virus that produces chicken pox) causes shingles, which would produce intense pain and a band of blisters on your back around your chest wall (along the nerve distribution). At times, it can seem like a heart attack, but the diagnosis is obvious to a doctor in most cases.

DIAGNOSING A HEART ATTACK

46. What is an electrocardiogram, and what is its diagnostic value?

An electrocardiogram (ECG or EKG) is the most important first test used to diagnose a heart attack. An ECG records the electrical activity of your heart through wires and electrodes attached to the skin of your arms, legs, and chest wall. Your heart's sinus node (Figure 4 and Question 4) generates electrical impulses that are recorded as wave patterns displayed on a monitor or are printed on paper (Figure 5). Since damaged heart muscle fails to conduct electrical impulses normally, the ECG may show an old (prior) heart attack or an acute (new) heart attack in progress.

The most important wave pattern in diagnosing a heart attack is the large Q wave (Figure 5) and the S-T segment elevation (ECG segment from the endpoint of the QRS complex to the beginning of the T wave; see Figure 5 and Question 4). When the entire thickness of your heart muscle is damaged, a large Q wave is shown on the ECG (then it's called a Q-wave myocardial infarction or a Q-wave heart attack). On the other hand, the term *non-Q-wave MI* is used when the ECG shows only an S-T segment change without the large Q wave. A non-Q-wave MI occurs when primarily the inner layer of your heart muscle is damaged.

When the ECG displays a large Q wave with the S-T segment elevation in a heart attack, the heart attack is considered to be acute, and the damage is in progress. As mentioned, a heart attack is considered to be old when there is a Q wave with no S-T segment elevation. Clinically, a Q-wave heart attack is said to be more serious than a non-Q-wave heart attack.

The ECG is also very important for diagnosing a variety of abnormal heart rhythms (cardiac arrhythmias; see Questions 57–67). In addition, the ECG provides extremely important information to your doctor in ruling out the diagnosis of a heart attack in dealing with various diseases and disorders that produce chest pain resembling that of a heart attack (see Questions 37–42).

47. What blood tests are available for diagnosing a heart attack?

Certain enzymes (protein molecules) normally found in the heart muscle leak out into the bloodstream when a heart attack damages the heart muscle. A blood test will show increased levels of these enzymes in the blood. (The blood test used most commonly to look for the presence of various enzymes is the measurement of CK-MB: creatine kinase myocardial band. (Our discussion here doesn't go into the technical explanation of the CK-MB marker.) Although CK-MB has been standard marker, it's not very accurate, since elevated levels can be found also in people without heart damage. Other enzymes may include troponins, myoglobin, and C-reactive protein.

48. Who needs a stress test? What is its diagnostic value?

Several different kinds of stress tests are used, but the test used most commonly is the treadmill stress test. Obviously, a stress test should not be performed when a heart attack is acute (i.e., in progress). The stress test is usually performed for screening or as a first-line evaluation of symptoms, particularly those of chest pain. This test evaluates how your heart and blood vessels respond to exertion; the results may indicate whether your chest pain is due to a coronary artery disease (CAD), particularly angina (see Question 10).

Stress test

test that evaluates how the heart and blood vessels respond to exertion and may allow diagnosis of coronary artery disease; may be performed using a treadmill or various chemicals (e.g., dobutamine, adenosine).

A **stress test** is essential for evaluating chest pain and marked shortness of breath, particularly that which is related to physical exercise. However, your doctor first would ensure against the probability of an acute (new) heart attack. The test is especially an important screening and diagnostic test for anyone with one or more coronary risk factors (see Question 16), even for those without a history of heart symptoms, including chest pain (see Question 30).

In a treadmill exercise stress test, you would walk on a motor-driven treadmill while a doctor monitors and records your ECG picture and your blood pressure (BP). During the test, your heart workload progressively increases until any significant symptom (e.g., chest pain) or some ECG abnormality develops. Every 3 minutes, a faster speed and an increase in the elevation (or slope) of the treadmill progressively increases your heart's workload.

If you are unable to walk on a treadmill, doctors can provide you with other forms of exercise, such as pedaling a stationary bicycle or performing arm exercises and various pharmacologic (nonexercise) stress tests. People with arthritis or other problems with walking can use such nonexercise stress tests as adenosine, dipyridamole, or dobutamine. These pharmacologic agents "stress" your heart (in the good sense of that term) by mimicking the effects of physical exercise.

Imaging tests provide useful additional diagnostic information by producing pictures of your heart during and after physical exercise or pharmacologic stress testing. Imaging tests may be used alone or may clarify the results of previous stress tests without using imaging.

49. What is a nuclear scan, and what is its diagnostic value?

A nuclear scan is a useful diagnostic test to identify problems of blood flow to your heart. Small amounts of radioactive material, such as thallium or a compound known as Cardiolyte, are injected into your bloodstream. Special cameras can detect the radioactive material as it flows through your heart and lungs; they can spot a decrease in blood supply to the heart muscle due to coronary artery disease.

50. What is an echocardiogram, and what is its diagnostic value?

An echocardiogram uses sound waves to produce an image of your heart. An echocardiogram machine directs sound waves at your heart through a wand-like device (called a transducer) held against your chest.

The sound waves bounce off your heart, reflect back through the chest wall, and proceeded electronically to produce video images of your heart on a monitor screen. An echocardiogram can identify an area of your heart muscle that's been damaged by a heart attack and can show the status of your heart's pumping action.

51. What is a coronary angiogram, and what is its diagnostic value?

Coronary angiogram (arteriogram)

x-ray study in which dye is used to demonstrate the degree and the location of coronary artery narrowing or blockage.

A **coronary angiogram** (**arteriogram**) is the definitive and most accurate diagnostic test for coronary artery disease. A coronary angiogram can precisely identify specific sites and degree of a narrowing (stenosis) or blockage of your coronary arteries. Therefore, a coronary angiogram is essential before any attempt to perform a coronary artery dilatation by coronary angioplasty (PTCA) or a coronary artery bypass surgery (see Question 77).

In a coronary angiogram, a doctor inserts a catheter (a long thin tube) into an artery in your groin area (or, less commonly, in your arm) and threads it through that artery to your heart arteries. Then the doctor injects a liquid dye into your coronary arteries by way of the catheter. As the dye (called contrast agent) flows through those coronary arteries, the doctor can accurately identify any narrowing (stenosis) and blockage of those arteries using a series of x rays and videotapes.

52. Are other tests available?

Several other tests are available for the diagnosis and treatment of coronary artery disease either directly or indirectly. The chest x ray can evaluate the condition of your lungs and the size and shape of your heart and major blood vessels. A chest x ray is particularly useful also for monitoring the management of various complications from a heart attack (see Questions 54 and 72).

Electron beam computerized tomography (EBCT), also called an ultrafast CT scan, scans your coronary arteries for signs of calcium within plaques that can cause coronary artery narrowing or blockage. When it detects a substantial amount of calcium, it almost certainly points to a diagnosis of coronary artery disease, because plaques contain some calcium in the majority of cases.

Magnetic resonance imaging (MRI) with enhanced software can provide accurate information about arterial blood flow, including that in very small coronary arteries not visible when using a coronary angiogram.

Electron beam computerized tomography (EBCT)

a new diagnostic test to detect calcium within plaques of coronary artery.

Magnetic resonance imaging (MRI)

a form of special diagnostic x-ray tests that can be used to diagnose coronary artery narrowing or blockage.

PART THREE

Problems After a Heart Attack

What are cardiac arrhythmias, and how should they be handled?

What is heart failure?

What is a heart block?

What is cardiac arrest?

More ...

53. What is ventricular wall rupture?

Ventricular wall rupture (rupture of the heart muscle of the ventricles) is the most serious and life-threatening complication of a heart attack. This is because the disorder causes rupture of the pumping chambers of the heart. As soon as the ventricles rupture, there will be no heart function at all, and sudden cardiac death is the immediate outcome. For nearly every patient who experiences ventricular wall rupture, there is no possible treatment.

54. What is congestive heart failure and what are its usual symptoms?

The heart muscle damage from a heart attack may be so extensive that the remaining heart muscle is unable to provide adequate pumping action. Consequently, blood flow to tissues and organs throughout the body (including the heart itself) markedly decreases, leading to congestion in the lungs and to a variety of symptoms and signs. This event is termed **congestive heart failure** (CHF) or simply **heart failure**.

Heart failure

inability of the heart to pump adequately; also called **congestive heart failure**.

Dyspnea

shortness of breath.

Edema

fluid accumulation resulting in swelling, commonly due to heart failure.

CHF displays various signs and symptoms. Shortness of breath (**dyspnea**), especially during physical exertion or upon lying down; fatigue and weakness; and **edema** (swelling) of the legs, ankles, and feet are symptoms characteristic of CHF. It also can lead to wheezing or coughing up white or pink blood-tinged phlegm (sputum); swelling of the abdomen and rapid weight gain from fluid retention; and engorged neck veins. Those experiencing CHF would have dizzy or fainting spells (syncope) and palpitations from abnormal heart rhythms (cardiac arrhythmias). Nausea and loss of appetite would also be evident. CHF can even cause diminished alertness and difficulty in concentrating.

55. What is cardiogenic shock?

Cardiogenic shock occurs after insufficient blood circulation to your body, including the heart muscle itself. It's the result of low and ineffective blood pressure (BP) brought on by a markedly diminished pumping action of the heart during or immediately after a heart attack. In cardiogenic shock, coronary arteries do not receive sufficient blood, so the heart becomes weaker, and the blood circulation further decreases. Unfortunately, this vicious cycle is fatal in most cases.

In 7 to 15% of cases, cardiogenic shock often occurs during the first few days after an acute heart attack. Cardiogenic shock tends to occur when 40% or more of the left ventricle is damaged by a heart attack, and advanced disease is often found in three major coronary arteries. Usually, cardiogenic shock is associated with advanced CHF in heart attack victims. (The scope of this book prevents discussion of the management of cardiogenic shock.)

56. What are cardiac arrhythmias and how should they be handled?

Various abnormal heart rhythms, known as **cardiac arrhythmias** (see Question 57), frequently occur after a heart attack damages the heart muscle. Abnormal heart rhythms may be benign (i.e., not harmful) and self-limited, but serious arrhythmias often lead to sudden death.

Problems After a Heart Attack

Cardiogenic shock
life-threatening complication of a heart attack, common signs of which include hypotension, clammy skin, unclear mental state, markedly reduced urine output, and very poor pumping action of the heart.

Cardiac arrhythmia
abnormal (slow, rapid, or irregular) heart rhythm.

Abnormal heart rhythms may be slow (called **brady-cardia** or **bradyarrhythmia**), fast (called **tachycardia** or **tachyarrthymia**), or irregular.

In most cases, if you were affected by this disorder you would need an **artificial cardiac pacemaker**, an electrical device that activates the heart with batteries, for a persisting slow heart rhythm (see Question 80). For rapid heart rhythms, on the other hand, your doctor could prescribe any of several medications (e.g., beta-blockers, calcium channel blockers, lidocaine, procainamide, amiodarone, and the like). To handle life-threatening rapid arrhythmia (ventricular fibrillation), your doctor would immediately apply electric shock (**defibrillation**; see Questions 84–86), the only life-saving measure. (See Question 57 for a detailed discussion of abnormal heart rhythms.)

Cardiac arrhythmia (also called cardiac dysrhythmia) may appear as too fast, too slow, or irregular heartbeats. Certain stimulants, such as stress, tobacco smoking, caffeine, and alcohol, can cause you to experience a variety of cardiac arrhythmias, even if you're apparently healthy. Under those circumstances, you wouldn't need any particular treatment other than eliminating or controlling the abovementioned stimulants. However, more than 4 million Americans suffer from recurrent or symptomatic arrhythmias that usually require treatment. Clinically, significant arrhythmias usually occur in older adults with coronary artery disease when the electrical system of the heart is disturbed.

Serious arrhythmias commonly are by-products of coronary artery disease damage to the heart, particularly that resulting from a heart attack. Life-threatening arrhythmia, particularly ventricular fibrillation,

---

Bradyarrhythmia

abnormally slow heart rhythm (also called **bradycardia**).

Tachyarrhythmia (or tachycardia)

rapid heart rhythm.

Artificial cardiac pacemaker

electrical device that activates the heart using batteries, used temporarily or implanted permanently.

Defibrillation

an electric shock applied to the chest to restore the regular heart rhythm.

must be terminated within a few minutes to prevent sudden death, especially in patients experiencing an acute heart attack.

57. Which arrhythmias are common?

A variety of common arrhythmias have been identified. **Ventricular fibrillation** (**VF**) is the most serious and life-threatening arrhythmia. In VF, the cardiac impulses arising from the ventricles (lower chambers) produce very fast, irregular and chaotic heart rhythm with no pumping action. Most people with VF become unconscious, and emergency treatment (medications, electrical shock, and CPR) must be provided immediately to prevent sudden death.

Premature beats or contractions are the heartbeats that occur earlier than the usual heart cycle and momentarily interrupt your heart's regular rhythm. **Atrial fibrillation** (**AF**) (see Question 62) causes your atria (the upper heart chambers) to beat very rapidly and chaotically. Your ventricles (the lower heart chambers) also beat rapidly at a rate of 120 to 160 beats per minute, which leads to an irregular and rapid heart rhythm. AF is very common among older adults, particularly those with diseased hearts. Atrial flutter also causes your atria to beat very rapidly, and your ventricles also beat rapidly but at a lesser rate (usually 125–175 beats per minute). Atrial flutter is not nearly as common as atrial fibrillation.

Superventricular tachycardia (SVT) is a fast and regular heart rhythm arising from your atria or AV node (Figure 4). In most cases, SVT begins and ends abruptly. People with **Wolff-Parkinson-White (WPW) syndrome** are born with an extra electrical pathway

Ventricular fibrillation (VF) is the most serious and life-threatening arrhythmia.

Atrial fibrillation (AF)

chaotic, irregular, and rapid cardiac rhythm arising from the atria.

Supraventricular

any location above the ventricles, namely in the atria or in the A-V node.

Tachyarrhythmia (or tachycardia)

rapid heart rhythm.

Wolff-Parkinson-White (WPW) syndrome

form of congenital anomaly that often causes a very rapid heart rhythm.

(called accessory pathway) between the atria and the ventricles. (This syndrome is named after three physicians who first described it.) In WPW syndrome, this extra pathway allows too many electrical impulses to reach the ventricles. That surplus of impulses can lead to a very rapid heart rhythm—up to 250–300 beats per minute in some cases.

Ventricular tachycardia (VT)

regular, rapid cardiac rhythm arising from the ventricles, a serious arrhythmia.

In **ventricular tachycardia** (VT), the heart impulses arising from the ventricles (lower heart chambers) produce a rapid heart rhythm (160–200 beats per minute). VT produces a broad (bizarre) QRS complex on an ECG (Figure 5). Ventricular tachycardia often deteriorates to ventricular fibrillation.

Heart block

slower-than-usual or absent conduction of the cardiac impulse from the atria to the ventricles. Also called **AV block.**

When **heart block** (or **AV block**) occurs, the electrical impulses from the atria (upper chambers of your heart) do not reach the ventricles (or lower chambers). This happens when a block occurs in the electrical conduction system (Figure 4), and it leads to slow heart rhythm. Your doctor would install an artificial pacemaker if such a block persisted or for symptomatic heart block (see Question 63).

Sick sinus syndrome

dysfunction of sinus node resulting in abnormally slow heart rhythm and leading to dizziness, near-syncope, or syncope.

Long Q-T syndrome

inherited medical disorder that often produces ventricular fibrillation and sudden death.

Sick sinus syndrome (SSS), a disorder of the sinus node (the natural pacemaker; see Figure 4) prevents the sinus node from producing sufficient heart impulses, leading to a slow heart rhythm (see Question 64). An artificial pacemaker is necessary for advanced SSS. Another syndrome, the **long Q-T syndrome**, is an inherited medical disorder. It often produces ventricular fibrillation and sudden death. In many cases, doctors treating patients with this syndrome would use certain medications, artificial pacemakers, and electrical shock treatment.

58. What are common signs and symptoms of arrhythmias?

Although arrhythmias may occur without producing symptoms at all, most people who have arrhythmias experience some symptoms and signs. Those symptoms and signs depend upon the nature and the type of arrhythmia.

Arrhythmias often cause palpitations, skipped heartbeats (premature beats), and a fluttering or pounding sensation in your chest. Then, too, you might feel racing or rapid heartbeats or, conversely, slowing of your heartbeats. Arrhythmias also cause irregular heartbeats.

Arrhythmias have been known to bring on chest discomfort or actual chest pain and shortness of breath (dyspnea). You might develop a periodic cough (usually from premature beats) and feel weak and fatigued. In addition, you might become light-headed or dizzy to the point of nearly fainting (near-syncope) or actually fainting (syncope). With extreme arrhythmias, you would lapse into unconsciousness (usually from ventricular fibrillation) or even die suddenly (from cardiac arrest or ventricular fibrillation).

59. What are common complications of arrhythmias?

When an arrhythmia is either very rapid or very slow and that pattern continues for a prolonged period, serious complications may occur. For example, if you were a victim of congestive heart failure (CHF), initially your heart would beat very quickly for a prolonged period. If that condition were not treated, your heart's pumping action would become inadequate, causing the CHF. On the other hand, CHF causes a variety of arrhythmias. Thus, the relationship between arrhythmia and CHF is bidirectional (i.e., it works both ways).

In certain arrhythmias, such as atrial fibrillation (AF), small blood clots tend to form in your heart. When these blood clots break loose and travel through your bloodstream to your brain, a stroke usually follows. Your chance of developing a stroke increases when you possess various coronary risk factors, such as high BP (see Questions 25 and 27).

When a very rapid or very slow heart rhythm significantly reduces blood circulation to your brain, you may develop fainting (syncope) or near-syncope. In a severe case, you would become unconscious.

Further, very rapid ventricular tachycardia (rapid and regular rhythm arising from the lower chambers), and particularly ventricular fibrillation (see Question 66), often cause sudden death unless treated promptly. Sudden cardiac death is very common among heart attack victims.

60. What tests can detect and diagnose various arrhythmias?

Many tests can detect and diagnose arrhythmias. An electrocardiogram (ECG or EKG) is a recording of the electrical events of your heart through wires and electrodes that doctors attach to the skin of your arms, legs, and chest wall. The ECG device records electrical events by displaying wave forms on a monitor or printing them on paper. Routine ECG tracing records these electrical events for 12 seconds, allowing your doctor to detect and diagnose various arrhythmias. When a routine ECG does not detect a suspected or expected arrhythmia, however, other diagnostic tests may be necessary (discussed shortly).

On the ECG paper, the initial small and round wave, called the P wave, represents the electrical stimulation of the atria (Figure 5). The tallest wave after the P wave is the QRS complex, which represents the stimulation of the ventricles. Another relatively large, triangular wave is the T wave; it represents the period when the ventricles "recharge" their electrical forces to be ready for the next stimulation. These electrical events in total represent one heart cycle, and the normal heart rhythm continues in a healthy heart (called normal sinus rhythm). When something disturbs the normal heart rhythm, various arrhythmias will occur.

An **ambulatory ECG** (or Holter monitor ECG, named after the scientist who invented it) is a continuous recording of the electrical events of your heart for 24 hours (sometimes up to 48–72) hours). The Holter monitor is small (about the size of a small camera). It's a portable ECG recorder, worn on a strap over your shoulder or around your waist. Several electrodes are attached to the skin on your chest, and they're connected by wires to the ECG recorder. You would be instructed to record any signs or symptoms in a diary that would match any such activities.

Ambulatory ECG test

noninvasive diagnostic test that records the electrical activity of the heart for 24 hours using a portable tape recorder to detect any abnormality of heart rhythm (also called a **Holter monitor**).

The Holter monitor ECG records continuously on tape (or on computer chips). When you return the monitor to your doctor's office or to the heart station of a hospital, a computer plays back and analyzes the tape and prints out the Holter monitor ECG diagnosis so a cardiologist can review it for a final diagnosis.

Event recorder

form of ambulatory ECG device that records only when an arrhythmia occurs.

The **event recorder** is another form of ambulatory ECG. It's similar to a Holter monitor ECG in that you would wear it for several days or weeks, but it's not for continuous recording. When any symptom occurs or when you feel what you think is an arrhythmia, you push a button, and the ECG records for 1 to 2 minutes. The event recorder is most useful for occasional arrhythmias.

Exercise ECG test

noninvasive diagnostic test for coronary artery disease using a motor-driven treadmill, bicycle, or certain chemicals. Also known as a **stress test**.

When any arrhythmia is considered to occur during physical exertion, a stress test (**exercise ECG test**) is very valuable. The most commonly used is a treadmill (monitor-driven) stress test. In a stress, or exercise ECG test, you walk on a treadmill (or ride a stationary bicycle) while a machine records an ECG of your heart's electrical activity. The stress test can reveal any exercise-related arrhythmia that may not be found during a resting ECG.

As described earlier, a stress test is extremely valuable for the evaluation of chest pain, particularly angina (see Question 48), but a stress test should not be performed when an acute heart attack is in progress or is strongly suspected.

Tilt table test

useful diagnostic tool to evaluate fainting spells (syncope or near-syncope).

The **tilt table test** is a useful diagnostic tool to evaluate fainting spells (syncope) or near-syncope that may result from certain arrhythmias. In this test, you would lie on a table that can be moved to almost an upright position while a doctor continuously monitors your ECG, BP, and symptoms. Of course, the tilt table test should not be performed when an acute heart attack is in progress.

When the abovementioned tests fail to disclose the necessary diagnostic and therapeutic information, doctors may perform an **electrophysiologic study** (EPS) to assess the exact nature of a difficult problem. Thus, an EPS is usually recommended for those with life-threatening arrhythmias, especially during or soon after an acute heart attack. The EPS is also used to detect and diagnose any suspected arrhythmias that are otherwise not detected.

During the EPS, a doctor inserts a special electrode catheter (a long, thin, flexible wire) into your veins and guides it into your heart. Using such catheters, doctors can identify the exact site causing a life-threatening arrhythmia. Thus, the EPS is very useful not only for the diagnosis of life-threatening arrhythmias but for proper management of a disorder.

61. What are premature beats?

Premature beats (contractions) are heartbeats that occur earlier than the underlying cardiac cycle and momentarily interrupt your heart rhythm. Premature beats may arise from the atria (then they're called atrial premature beats) or from the ventricles (in which case they're called ventricular premature beats). They're the most common arrhythmias. Premature beats may occur in healthy people, but they occur more frequently in those with various heart diseases. It can be said that almost all adults experience premature beats from time to time. Some people don't even know it, but most experience some unpleasant feelings, such as "skipped heartbeats" or "funny sensation in the chest."

By and large, healthy people don't need active treatment for occasional premature beats other than avoiding possible stimulants, such as caffeine. On the other hand, patients with active heart disease, particularly a heart

Electrophysiologic study

insertion of a special electrode catheter into the veins and from there into the heart to identify the exact site causing life-threatening arrhythmias.

Almost all adults experience premature beats from time to time.

Problems After a Heart Attack

attack, need active treatment when ventricular premature beats occur very frequently in certain patterns (e.g., multiformed, meaning a different pattern in each premature beat). Under these circumstances, frequent ventricular premature beats may be considered a potential warning sign for more serious arrhythmias, such as ventricular tachycardia or fibrillation (see Question 65).

62. What is atrial fibrillation?

Atrial fibrillation (AF) occurs when electrical impulses arise from multiple sites in the atria (upper chambers) in a chaotic and uncoordinated fashion. Thus, the atrial wall can't squeeze the blood down to the ventricles. Only some of the rapid atrial impulses travel down to the ventricles because the atrial impulses must slow down in the AV node (Figure 4), which acts as a "relay station." The resulting irregular and usually (although not always) rapid heart rhythm is typical of AF.

When AF occurs, like most people you would experience some uncomfortable feelings: fluttering or pounding in your chest, weakness, light-headedness, shortness of breath, and chest discomfort with actual chest pain. The major concern is the increased risk for developing a stroke in people with recurrent or longstanding AF. AF tends to produce blood clots within the heart because of ineffective atrial contraction. Such blood clots may cause a blockage of the arteries in the brain, and that can cause a stroke.

Various medications are available to restore normal heart rhythm or at least to control rapid heart rate brought on by AF. Some people require electrical shock treatment to terminate AF (see Question 84). **Anticoagulants** (blood-thinning medications) are rec-

Anticoagulants

medications that interfere with or prevent blood clot formation.

ommended for treating patients with recurrent or chronic AF to prevent a potential stroke.

63. What is a heart block?

A heart block (atrioventricular or AV block) is an interruption of the heart impulses from the atria (commonly the sinus node) to the ventricles. This interruption results from a conduction block that occurs within the AV node and other conduction pathways (e.g., the His bundle and other branches; see Figure 4). Although the conduction interruption can be either partial (incomplete) or complete, discussion deals with **complete heart block** because of its clinical importance.

In complete heart block, all heart impulses from the atria are blocked, and none of them reach the ventricles. Consequently, a "backup pacemaker" (usually the AV node or the ventricles themselves) stimulates the ventricles. Thus, the heart rhythm in a heart block is very slow and unstable (a rate of 25–40 beats per minute). Heart block often produces various symptoms such as light-headedness, a fainting spell (syncope), and weakness. In addition, heart block may cause CHF or may worsen preexisting CHF (see Question 54). An artificial pacemaker is needed for persisting heart block (see Question 87).

Complete heart block

disturbance of normal conduction from the atria to the ventricles preventing electrical impulses from traveling through the heart muscle and conduction system, causing a very slow heart rhythm.

64. What is sick sinus syndrome?

Sick sinus syndrome (SSS) is a disorder in which the sinus node (the natural pacemaker; see Figure 4) fails to produce sufficient heart impulses. That failure leads to an unstable and slow heart rhythm. At times, slow heart rhythm may be mixed with rapid heart rhythms (e.g., in AF or ventricular tachycardia). That combination of slow and rapid heart rhythm is called the bradycardia-tachycardia syndrome.

Various symptoms (almost the same as those in a heart block) may be observed in advanced SSS. An artificial pacemaker is needed to treat advanced SSS, and additional medications may be necessary to treat the tachycardia (rapid rhythm) part of this disorder.

65. What is ventricular tachycardia?

Ventricular tachycardia (VT) is a rapid and regular heart rhythm (140–180 beats per minute) with bizarre (broad) QRS complexes (Figure 5). The impulses arise from the ventricles (lower heart chambers), commonly in an area of the heart muscle damaged by a heart attack. VT may occur suddenly for a short period and may stop without treatment.

However, VT often lasts for a long time, especially in the setting of an acute heart attack. It may deteriorate into a more serious arrhythmia: ventricular fibrillation (discussed in Question 66). VT may cause a variety of symptoms, such as light-headedness (near-syncope), fainting (syncope), shortness of breath, weakness, chest pain, and a feeling of impending death.

A physician would use various medications (e.g., lidocaine, amiodarone, procainamide, and the like) to treat and prevent VT. In some cases, when drug management is not effective, a physician might resort to the use of electrical shock treatment (**direct-current shock**). When VT persists or recurs, an electrophysiologic study (EPS, discussed in Question 60) can determine the exact nature of VT, and then the physician can arrange

Direct-current shock

electric shock for rapid heart rhythm.

for more effective management. Selected cases may require an **implantable cardioverter-defibrillator** (see Question 86) to control recurrent and serious VT.

66. What is ventricular fibrillation?

Ventricular fibrillation is an uncoordinated, irregular, and very rapid heart rhythm arising from multiple sites within the ventricles. VF is the most serious and life-threatening arrhythmia because it prevents any pumping action. Consequently, it stops any blood circulation in your entire body, and you lose consciousness instantly. Death follows within a few minutes unless emergency treatment restores your normal heart rhythm. Such emergency treatment can include CPR, electrical cardiac defibrillation, and the like (see Questions 68–73).

When emergency treatment is delayed for more than 4 minutes, damage to the brain may become permanent, even if a stable heart rhythm is restored later. Thus, immediate emergency treatment for VF is essential.

67. What is cardiac arrest?

Cardiac arrest is the stopping of any heart pumping action. Naturally, that means that all blood circulation to the entire body stops as well. Cardiac arrest is by no means any particular heart rhythm diagnosis. The underlying arrhythmia that most commonly causes cardiac arrest is ventricular fibrillation (discussed in Question 66), especially in those who experience acute heart attacks. Occasionally, the lack of any electrical activity at all in the heart can cause cardiac arrest. In addition, the disorder may be due to other extremely slow and ineffective heart rhythms.

Implantable cardioverter-defibrillator (ICD)

small electronic device implanted in the chest to deliver an electrical shock automatically when ventricular fibrillation or tachycardia develops.

Problems After a Heart Attack

From a clinical standpoint, cardiac arrest usually occurs together with pulmonary arrest (absence of lung function, which prevents effective breathing). This combination can lead to what you've heard described as cardiopulmonary arrest (the absence of both heart and lung function at the same time). As in cases of ventricular fibrillation, emergency treatment for cardiac or cardiopulmonary arrest (e.g., CPR, electrical cardioversion, and the like) is essential.

PART FOUR

Treating a Heart Attack

What medications are commonly used
for heart attack victims?

What is thrombolytic therapy, and who needs it?

What is coronary angioplasty, and who needs it?

What is a coronary stent, and who needs it?

More . . .

68. What are the general guidelines for heart attack management?

Patient comment:

When you feel as though you are having a heart attack, you should stop all of physical activity at once and lie or sit down. You or a person nearby—a friend or family member, or even a passing stranger with a cell phone if necessary— should call 911 for immediate medical attention; it is important that you get to the nearest hospital emergency room quickly. However, you should never drive your own car—that's far more dangerous than simply waiting for the ambulance, because if you become unconscious, you could wind up in an accident, possibly killing yourself and maybe even someone else. Even when you are not sure whether you are having a heart attack, if you know you have high risk for heart attacks, it's better to over-diagnose (or overreact) than to respond too late to the real thing. Do not hesitate to call 911 even if you wonder whether it is only a false alarm.

Cardiopulmonary resuscitation (CPR)
life-saving technique using artificial respiration and cardiac massage to restore normal functions of the heart and lungs after cardiac arrest.

Immediate **cardiopulmonary resuscitation** (CPR) and direct-current shock (defibrillation) are essential for your survival of sudden cardiac death (see Questions 84–86 and Question 90). As soon as a heart attack occurs, either you or your family members or friends should dial 911 to request an ambulance. The 911 dispatcher will contact the emergency medical services (EMS) system. When the 911 system is not available, you or others should contact the emergency medical response system in the local area. The EMS responders should reach you within 4 to 5 minutes. As time permits, you or others acting for you should also inform your family (private) physician.

If you are conscious, you should chew one regular-strength aspirin—chew it, don't just swallow it, because chewing it will speed up its absorption. Studies have shown that taking aspirin while an acute heart attack is in progress can reduce the death rate by 25%. Aspirin is effective in inhibiting blood clotting, so taking it improves and maintains blood flow through a narrowed heart artery, which can make the difference between life and death in some patients.

You should stop all physical actions and situate yourself, or have others situate you, in the most comfortable body position (lying or sitting). You could take nitroglycerin (up to three tablets) under your tongue *if it has been prescribed before* for angina. Do not take someone else's nitroglycerin on the assumption that it will help—it might make matters worse! If you were found unconscious, as soon as is possible any family member or friend trained in administering CPR—and certainly the responding paramedical personnel—should initiate CPR. As you are being transported by an ambulance to a nearby hospital emergency room (ER), those in the EMS team will provide this emergency treatment as needed until you are stable. They should also give you any available emergency cardiac drugs promptly as needed. And, of course, continuous medical care will be provided in the ER.

Do not try to deny what is happening in such circumstances; avoiding the truth can literally be fatal to heart attack victims. And you should avoid self-diagnosis or self-treatment (this is especially true for someone who might be a physician). It goes without saying that you shouldn't be driving in this condition; again, don't try to get yourself to the hospital, call an ambulance instead.

Early diagnosis followed by effective early medical care is extremely important for a better chance of survival

Taking aspirin while an acute heart attack is in progress can reduce the death rate by 25%.

Avoiding the truth can literally be fatal to heart attack victims.

Treating a Heart Attack

and a good outcome. As soon as you are examined in the ER and undergo necessary diagnostic tests, the most important treatment is **thrombolytic therapy** (the use of special mediations that dissolve blood clots). These agents will reperfuse (i.e., restore circulation) in the damaged heart muscle (see Question 70). Other medications also will are discussed in Questions 69 and 70.

The management of acute heart attack is carried out primarily by five major modalities as follows:

- Various medications
- Electrical shock treatment (defibrillation) and artificial pacemaker (see Question 80–88)
- Coronary angioplasty (percutaneous transluminal coronary angioplasty or PTCA, see Questions 72–76)
- Coronary artery bypass graft (CABG, see Questions 77 and 78)
- Cardiopulmonary resuscitation (CPR, see Question 90 in Part Five)

For ventricular fibrillation (chaotic, irregular and ineffective rapid heart rhythm arising from the ventricles, see Questions 57 and 66), electric shock should be applied immediately using automatic external defibrillators (AEDs, see Question 85). Otherwise, sudden death cannot be prevented in most cases. Most ambulance teams carry portable defibrillators, and many police and fire rescue units are also equipped with defibrillators. AEDs are very simple to operate and are also available in some commercial airplanes and public places (e.g., large sports fields, music halls, and convention auditoriums). AEDs are often lifesaving devices for heart attack victims before reaching the hospital ER.

Thrombolytic therapy

intravenous administration of medications that dissolve blood clots blocking the coronary arteries.

If you were experiencing chest pain, the attending physician might administer various commonly used narcotics (painkillers, such as morphine) and would give you oxygen, usually a part of management. In addition, nitroglycerin is often used, because it temporarily opens up narrowed arteries, improving blood flow to your heart muscle.

When the emergency treatment is completed in the ER, those in attendance would transfer you to the coronary (cardiac) care unit (CCU) for further management along with more diagnostic tests (see Questions 46–52). After they fully evaluated you in the CCU, they would attempt coronary angioplasty (dilatation of narrowed or blocked coronary arteries; see Question 72) after a coronary angiogram (see Question 51).

If you did not respond satisfactorily to coronary angioplasty (another term for percutaneous transluminal coronary angioplasty, or PCTA) or those attending you found it to be technically difficult, they would consider a coronary artery bypass graft (CABG; see Question 77).

69. What medications are commonly used to treat heart attack victims?

There are many medications used in the treatment of a heart attack, but the most important medications are various thrombolytic agents (medications to dissolve the blood clots in the coronary arteries). Thrombolytic therapy is discussed in detail in Question 70).

Commonly used agents are digoxin (often called heart pill), beta-blockers, angiotensin-converting enzyme (ACE) inhibitors, diuretics (often called water pills), angiotensin II receptor blockers, and spironolactone (Aldacton). The scope of this book does not permit detailed discussion of these medications.

When these medications are not effective, various medical/surgical devices, such as a heart pump (called left ventricular assist devices), a biventricular artificial cardiac pacemaker (see Question 80), and even an artificial heart have been used in the management of advanced CHF. In addition, the treatment of the underlying coronary artery disease such as coronary artery dilatation (coronary angioplasty, see Question 72) and coronary artery bypass surgery (see Question 77) is very important in the management of CHF. When all of this management is not effective, the transplantation of a new heart must be considered as a last resort in the treatment of far-advanced CHF. When advanced CHF fails to improve in heart attack victims, a fatal outcome is often unavoidable.

An additional medication is found in the common aspirin. Heart attack victims are advised to chew one regular-strength aspirin when first experiencing chest discomfort. Aspirin is effective in inhibiting blood clotting in the coronary arteries. ER personnel often use "super aspirin" (a platelet II-*b*/III-*a* receptor blocker) together with a thrombolytic agent. Super aspirin has been found to be more potent than regular aspirin in preventing new blood clot formation. Anticoagulants (blood-thinning drugs), such as heparin or hirudin, often can prevent blood clotting. The relief of chest pain usually requires various narcotics (painkillers), such as morphine. Additionally, doctors commonly use nitroglycerin to relieve chest pain because this drug temporarily opens up narrowed coronary arteries and improves blood flow to the heart muscle.

Various beta-blocking medications are effective in lowering rapid heart rates and blood pressure so that the workload of the damaged heart muscle can be reduced. **Anti-arrhythmic agents** include various medications (e.g., lidocaine, procainamide, amiodarone) needed to manage and prevent a variety of rapid heart rhythms (see Questions 56 and 65).

Lipid or cholesterol-lowering drugs (e.g., statins, niacin) will reduce blood cholesterol. They're beneficial if given early after a heart attack for a better chance of survival. The management of various complications (e.g., CHF, cardiogenic shock, as discussed in Question 55) requires many other medications (e.g., digoxin, antihypertensive drugs).

Anti-arrhythmic agents

medications such as quinidine or procainamide (Pronestyl) used for the prevention and treatment of various cardiac arrhythmias.

70. What is thrombolytic therapy and when is it used?

Patient comment:

When you suffer from a heart attack, the most important medication is thrombolytic agent (a drug to dissolve blood clots blocking your heart arteries). This thrombolytic agent is most effective when given within 30 minutes to 3 hours after the onset of a heart attack. That's why you should not delay seeking medical attention as soon as you feel like you are having a heart attack. If the agent is given more than 24 hours after the beginning of the symptoms, it does you almost no good at all.

Table 1 Drugs commonly used in the treatment of heart attack and related disorders

Type	Generic Name	Brand Name	Manufacturer
Thrombolytic	Alteplase	Activase®	Genentech
Thrombolytic	Retoplase	Retevase	Boehringer
Thrombolytic	Urokinase	Abbokinase®	Abbott
Thrombolytic	Streptokinase	Streptase®	Aventis
Anticoagulant	Aspirin	Bayer, Anacin Excedrin	Bayer Wyeth Consumer Bristol-Myers Squibb
Anticoagulant	Clopidogrel bisulfate	Plavix®	Sanofi-Sythelabo
Anticoagulant	Heparin		Wyeth-Ayerst
Anticoagulant	Warfarin	Coumadin®	Bristol-Myers Squibb
Antianginal	Nitroglycerin	Nitro-bid®	Hoechst
Beta blocker	Carvedilol	Coreg®	GlaxoSmithKline
Beta blocker	Metoprolol	Lopressor®	Novartis
Beta blocker	Nadolol	Corgard®	Bristol-Myers Squibb
Beta blocker	Propanolol	Inderal®	Wyeth-Ayerst
Anti-arrhythmic	Procainamide	Procanbid®	Parke-Davis
Anti-arrhythmic	Lidocaine	Xylocaine®	Astra-Zeneca
Anti-arrhythmic	Amiodarone	Cordarone®	Wyeth-Ayerst
Anti-arrhythmic	Phenytoin	Dilantin®	Parke-Davis
Anti-arrhythmic (also inotropic)	Digoxin	Lanoxin®	GlaxoSmithKline
Anti-arrhythmic	Diltiazem	Cardizem®	Biovail
Cholesterol-lowering	Atorvastatin	Lipitor®	Pfizer
Cholesterol-lowering	Lovastatin	Mevacor®	Merck
Cholesterol-lowering	Pravastatin	Pravachol®	Bristol-Myers Squibb
Cholesterol-lowering	Simvastatin	Zocor®	Merck
Diuretic	Spironolactone	Aldactone®	Searle
Antihypertensive	Benazepril	Lotensin©	Novartis
Antihypertensive	Lisinopril	Zestril	Astra-Zeneca
Antihypertensive	Amlodipine	Norvasc®	Pfizer
Antihypertensive	Diltiazem	Cardizemr®	Biovail
Antihypertensive	Nifedipine	Procardia®	Pfizer
Antihypertensive	Enalapril	Vasotec®	Merck

Thrombolytic therapy is the intravenous administration of medications that dissolve blood clots blocking your coronary arteries. The thrombolytic agents are often called **clot busters**. The earlier you receive a thrombolytic agent after a heart attack, the greater your chance of survival. That's because reducing the damage of your heart muscle leads to improved pumping action. Thus, thrombolytic therapy is a mainstay in the early management of heart attack at the present time.

For best therapeutic results, the thrombolytic agent must be administered within 30 minutes to 3 hours after the onset of symptoms. Giving the agent later than 3 hours reduces the beneficial effects of thrombolytic therapy. Delaying such treatment for 12 to 24 hours drastically reduces the therapy's beneficial effects. In addition, if the agent is administered after more than 24 hours from the onset of symptoms, thrombolytic therapy produces little or no beneficial effect.

At present, the most important and standard thrombolytic drug is tPA or alteplase (Activase) in the United States. The next most commonly used thrombolytic agents are retoplase (Retavase), urokinase (Abbokinase), and finally streptokinase (Kabikinase, Streptase). In addition, other thrombolytic agents may include lanoteplase, anistreplase, and tenectoplase (the newest drug).

A thrombolytic drug, most commonly alteplase, is given intravenously with an anticoagulant agent (e.g., heparin). Heparin and aspirin are unable to destroy existing blood clots, but they can prevent blood clots from reforming after they are broken up.

Clot busters
another term for thrombolytic agents, medications that dissolve blood clots.

The earlier you receive a thrombolytic agent after a heart attack, the greater is your chance of survival.

Treating a Heart Attack

Certain limitations govern who the best candidates are for thrombolytic therapy. For example, you would have had to experience symptoms of acute heart attack within 3 hours after their onset (within 12 hours at most). Also, if you are an adult younger than 75 years and have an S-T segment elevation on an ECG (Figure 5 and Question 46), you are considered a good candidate. If as a heart attack victim you had a systolic BP of less than 180 mm Hg, any heart rate, and diabetes, you would qualify.

In some clinical circumstances, your doctor would avoid thrombolytic therapy or use it with great caution. If you were older than 75 years, you'd be at a higher risk, even if you were otherwise in good general health. Then, too, such therapy would not be used if your heart attack symptoms had continued for more than 12 hours. The same precaution would apply to you if you were pregnant. Your doctor might hesitate to use thrombolytic therapy, or use it cautiously, if your ECG demonstrated no S-T segment elevation (see Question 46 and Figure 5), even if the diagnosis of a new heart attack were certain.

Others who would prompt caution are those with recent trauma (especially head injury) or surgery, heart attack victims recovered from prolonged CPR (see Question 90), and those with active peptic ulcers.

Thrombolytic therapy would *not* be used at all in treating those with recent major bleeding from any organ or for those whose ECG demonstrated a depressed S-T segment (Figure 5), such as seen in a non–Q wave heart attack. Doctors would avoid using such therapy also for treating people with a history of stroke, particularly **cerebral hemorrhage**, and those with uncontrolled and extremely elevated high BP.

As long as the above-mentioned conditions are not present, thrombolytic therapy should be considered as the first-line lifesaving measure for any heart attack victim, regardless of age or gender.

71. Does thrombolytic therapy produce complications?

Fortunately, complications and side effects from thrombolytic therapy are rare. Hemorrhagic stroke (cerebral hemorrhage) is the most serious complication of thrombolytic therapy, and it usually occurs during the first day after the administration of the agent. The chances of this occurring are reported to be 0.5 to 0.1%. In addition, internal bleeding may occur in other organs, such as the intestines, stomach, and urinary tracts. Other side effects may be allergic reactions to the agents, hypotension (low BP), and **cholesterol embolization**.

Streptokinase (one of the thrombolytic agents) given without heparin is reported to show the lowest risk of complication. However, its effectiveness in restoring blood flow is less than that of other thrombolytic agents. The mortality (death) rate from bleeding is reported to be 3 in every 1,000 patients treated with thrombolytic therapy, but its survival benefits, particularly in combination with aspirin, last for many years.

Other aspects of managing a heart attack include percutaneous transluminal coronary angioplasty (PTCA),

Cerebral hemorrhage

a form of stroke with hemorrhage (bleeding) in the brain.

Cholesterol embolization

cholesterol clot formation in the bloodstream.

Treating a Heart Attack

coronary artery bypass graft (CABG), an artificial pacemaker, electric shock treatment, and cardiopulmonary resuscitation (CPR). Another new device called an atherectomy catheter can shave off and remove plaque from the inside of the diseased coronary artery. A new device called a laser-tipped catheter can vaporize the blockage of the diseased coronary artery with a tiny laser beam. This new device may be useful when the blocked or narrowed segment of the diseased coronary artery is long, and the ordinary PTCA is technically difficult to perform. These therapeutic modalities are discussed in detail in Questions 78 to 82.

72. What is coronary angioplasty, and who needs it?

Percutaneous transluminal coronary angioplasty (PTCA)

standard revascularization procedure to open up narrowed or blocked coronary arteries.

Coronary angioplasty (an abbreviated term for **percutaneous transluminal coronary angioplasty** or PTCA) is one of two standard revascularization procedures to open up the narrowed (stenotic) or blocked coronary arteries. Emergency coronary angioplasty is the more commonly performed procedure for practically all heart attack patients. Coronary angioplasty is most successful when performed within 12 hours after the onset of symptoms, and the sooner the better. A cardiac surgical team must be available immediately in case the PTCA is unsuccessful and produces major complications (discussed shortly).

After injecting a local anesthetic into the groin (less frequently in the arm), doctors place a narrow tube (catheter) containing a fiber optic camera and direct it to the narrowed or blocked coronary artery. Then they pass a tiny deflated balloon through the catheter to the narrowed or blocked coronary artery as they watch an x-ray image on a TV screen. They advance the guide catheter in the diseased coronary artery until it arrives at the blockage. At that point, they inject a small amount of contrast material through the catheter, watching the procedure on the screen, to determine the exact location of the blockage or narrowing of the coronary artery.

They then inflate the small balloon to squeeze the plaque against the walls of the coronary artery. That action flattens out the plaque and opens up the narrowed artery so that it will be able to restore blood circulation. The doctors inflate the balloon for perhaps 30 to 120 seconds and then deflate it. Chest pain often occurs when the balloon is inflated because the blood flow is temporarily interrupted by the balloon in the segment of the heart muscle. Medical staff should be informed as soon as a brief chest pain occurs. They inflate and deflate the balloon several times thereafter.

Doctors sometimes use a relatively new device called a **coronary stent**, an expandable metal mesh tube. They commonly implant the stent during PTCA—about 80% of angioplasty procedures—at the site of the blockage to prevent restenosis of the coronary artery.

Coronary stent
expandable metal mesh tube used in PTCA to prevent restenosis of the coronary artery.

When the PTCA is considered to be successful, doctors remove the balloon catheter and perform a coronary angiogram (visualization of coronary arteries by movie camera) to assess the improved coronary blood circulation. Then they remove the guide catheter. Most patients are able to go home by 1 to 2 days after the procedure.

73. How do I prepare for coronary angioplasty?

Unless you were already hospitalized, you would be admitted to the hospital on the day of the procedure or on the night before. You would be told not to eat or drink anything after midnight (at least 6–8 hours before the procedure). When the hospital staff were certain that you understood the procedure (its purpose, potential benefits, and possible risks), you would sign a consent form.

Before the procedure, after routine blood tests, the staff would perform an electrocardiogram (ECG) and a chest x ray. They would clean and shave your groin area (or your arm area in some cases) to prevent any infection before inserting the catheters (also as a part of the procedure). They would insert a small intravenous needle (IV line) into an arm vein for administering fluids and medications as needed. It would be a good idea to empty your bladder as completely as possible before the procedure starts. (Of course, a bedpan or urinal would be available during the procedure).

74. What is a coronary stent, and when is it used?

A coronary stent is a relatively new device implanted permanently in the diseased coronary artery to keep the diseased coronary artery open during and after coronary angioplasty. It is used in up to 60 to 80% of patients who undergo PTCA. The stent is a fine-slotted, metallic coil, tube, or mesh structure inserted into the diseased coronary artery at the site where PTCA procedure dilated the blocked or narrowed coronary artery. The stent can reduce various complications, such as a new heart attack or a restenosis of the coronary artery. Research has shown that the restenosis rate after a simple coronary angioplasty without a stent is 30 to 40%, but the restenosis rate is reduced to 20% when a stent is used. Thus, the stent is used practically for every patient who undergoes coronary angioplasty.

The coronary stent is mounted on a balloon catheter and delivered to the site of severe narrowing or blockage of the coronary artery. When the balloon is inflated, the stent expands and is pressed against the inner wall of the diseased coronary artery. After the balloon is deflated and removed, the coronary stent permanently remains in place to prevent restenosis.

Several different kinds of stents are produced in various designs, but the most commonly used stent is the Palmaz-Shatz stent. This stent is a small, slotted, stainless-steel tube about half an inch long, and it weighs as little as a straight pin. It is as narrow as a piece of thin noodle. One or more coronary stents may be used in the coronary artery when the narrowed or blocked segment of the artery is long. New tissue will slowly grow over the stent within a few weeks and will completely cover the stent.

75. What medications are commonly used during and after coronary angioplasty?

Restenosis of the coronary artery during or shortly after a successful coronary angioplasty is often (but not always) due to blood clots. Doctors frequently use anticlotting agents (medications to prevent blood clots), such as aspirin, heparin, coumarin, or combinations of these drugs, during and after the coronary angioplasty to prevent restenosis. Actually, aspirin is found to be more effective than heparin for this purpose.

New anticlotting agents, such as tirofiban or clopidogrel, may be effective in preventing restenosis when they are administered in combination with heparin or aspirin. However, in some cases, restenosis of the diseased coronary artery cannot be prevented by using the above-mentioned anticlotting drugs during or after angioplasty. That's because restenosis in some cases is due to unknown causes.

76. What are the potential risks involved with coronary angioplasty?

The risks from coronary angioplasty are generally minimal, and its significant benefits usually outweigh the risks in treating heart attack patients. Potential risks involved with coronary angioplasty may include tearing or cracking of the coronary artery lining, which might close the treated artery, or cause a new heart attack or stroke or even (rarely) death. Because of such risks from coronary angioplasty, a cardiac surgical team must stand by during an angioplasty.

77. What is a coronary artery bypass graft, and when is it used?

A coronary artery bypass graft (CABG) is the major cardiac surgery performed most commonly in America and in all other civilized countries worldwide. CABG may be performed as an emergency operation, but it is performed more commonly as an elective surgery. Surgeons perform it when coronary angioplasty or thrombolytic therapy (discussed earlier in Questions 70 and

71) is not successful or is not appropriate. When CABG is scheduled (rather than as an emergency surgery), they usually do this a few days later to allow recovery of the heart muscle. A recent study showed that 1-year risk of death is reduced by more than 40% when coronary angioplasty or CABG is performed within 14 days after the onset of acute heart attack. The PTCA is initially successful in more than 90% of cases.

A CABG makes a bypass (detour) to reestablish blood circulation around the blocked segment of the coronary artery (Figure 9). Most commonly, a saphenous vein obtained from the leg is installed as a bypass vessel so that blood flow around the blockage from the aorta (the largest arterial trunk) to the coronary artery will be established (Figure 9). Less commonly, one or

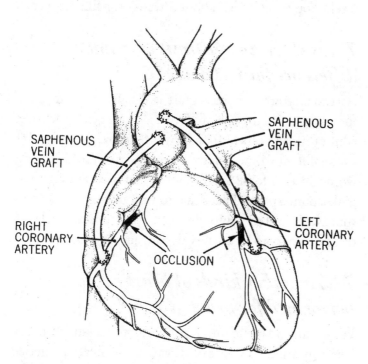

SAPHENOUS VEIN GRAFT

SAPHENOUS VEIN GRAFT

RIGHT CORONARY ARTERY

LEFT CORONARY ARTERY

OCCLUSION

Figure 9   Coronary artery bypass surgery.

both internal mammary arteries (arteries in the chest wall, normally arising from branches of the aorta) are used for a CABG.

Doctors commonly perform a CABG to relieve a blocked left main coronary artery (Figure 9); a diffusely narrowed or blocked coronary artery; a disease involving multiple coronary arteries; and poor function of the left ventricle. In addition, a CABG also helps to overcome significant technical difficulty during PTCA, when PTCA is unsuccessful, and when there are serious complications during PTCA. Such complications might include rupture of the coronary artery, worsening of the blockage, and the occurrence of a new heart attack.

After a CABG, you would stay in the hospital for 1 week. You would need about 3 weeks for full recovery.

78. Is there an age limit or gender difference for CABG?

A coronary artery bypass graft is usually recommended for adults up to the age of 75 years. However, some older adults (80–85 years old) underwent CABG recently with successful outcomes. The outcome of CABG among women seems to be less favorable than that among their male counterparts. That's due to various reasons, such as some technical difficulty during CABG and the delayed diagnosis of coronary artery disease among women.

79. Are other kinds of heart surgery performed for heart attacks?

When any major complications of heart attack occur (see Questions 53 to 60), a variety of heart surgeries might be necessary. In the event of mitral regurgitation (leaking back of blood flow from the left ventricle to the left atrium because of mitral valve dysfunction; see Figure 2), physicians would replace the mitral valve with an artificial heart valve. When an acute heart attack produces a **ventricular septal defect** (formation of a hole in the ventricular septum between two ventricles; see Figure 2), a surgeon would repair the hole immediately.

When a major complication, such as congestive heart failure (markedly diminished pumping action of the heart; see Questions 53–57), persists or deteriorates in spite of all available therapy, you would need transplantation of a new heart or an artificial heart (see Question 80).

80. What is an artificial pacemaker, and when is it used?

When medications and varied medical or surgical treatments are not effective or appropriate, the resolution of certain medical conditions requires electrical treatment. One of two major electrical devices or methods is an artificial pacemaker (Figure 10). The other is the use of electrical shocks. An artificial pacemaker is a small, battery-operated device that regulates your heartbeat by imitating your natural heart rhythm arising from the sinus node (your natural pacemaker). Some artificial pacemakers are permanent units (internal) implanted in the chest; others are temporary (external) units.

Most artificial pacemakers have a sensing device that turns off when your natural heart rhythm is faster than the preset desired heart rate, and it turns back on when your heart rate becomes slower than that preset rate.

Ventricular septal defect

hole (abnormal communication) in the muscle wall between the ventricles, a common form of congenital heart disease and possibly caused by a heart attack; a life-threatening complication.

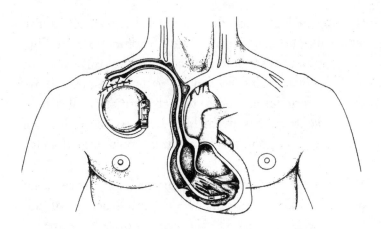

Figure 10 Artificial cardiac pacemaker in the body.

This type of artificial pacemaker is called a demand pacemaker. At present, almost all pacemakers are manufactured as demand pacemakers.

The artificial pacemaker consists of two parts: the pulse generator and wires (insulated leads). The pulse generator is a small metal "can" that contains a battery and electrical circuitry (a computer). They regulate the rate of electrical impulses sent to your heart. The pulse generator is implanted in your chest, just below your collarbone in most cases (Figure 10). However, for cosmetic reasons, physicians can implant the pulse generator elsewhere (e.g., in the area between the upper chest wall and arm, or the armpit).

Newer models are much smaller and lighter than older models. The smaller models weigh less than an ounce and are about the size of three silver dollars sandwiched together. Their battery life is generally 6 to 7 years, but batteries may operate for up to 10 to 12 years. The pulse generator must be replaced periodically before the pacemaker batteries wear out.

A surgeon threads the pacemaker wires (insulated leads) through a large vein and into the heart, and these flexible wires are connected to the pulse generator. Thus, these wires deliver the electrical impulses from the pulse generator to the heart.

Managing various slow heart rhythms primarily requires an artificial pacemaker, particularly for significant symptoms, such as dizziness and near-syncope or syncope, associated with these abnormal rhythms (see Questions 57 to 60). Occasionally, treatment of advanced congestive heart failure (markedly diminished pumping action of the heart) also requires an artificial pacemaker (see Question 53).

Certain medical conditions require the use of an artificial pacemaker. For example, in the sick sinus syndrome, your natural pacemaker (the sinus node) is unable to produce sufficient heart impulses; that creates a very slow and unstable heart rhythm (see Question 57). In this disorder, slow heart rhythm often coexists with components of very rapid rhythms, such as atrial fibrillation or ventricular tachycardia. That leads to a combination of slow and rapid heart rhythms (called bradytachycardia; see Question 64).

In another condition, heart block (AV block), the interruption in conducting your heart impulse to your ventricles (lower chambers) causes a very slow heart rhythm. This interruption is the result of a block in the conduction system, commonly in the AV node (Figure 4 and Question 63).

Physicians may use biventricular pacemakers in some cases of advanced congestive heart failure. That's the case when all available medications are not effective enough to relieve congestive heart failure (see Question 53). Biventricular pacemakers stimulate both the right and the left ventricles in a coordinated fashion so that the pumping action can be improved.

81. Are different pacing methods used?

In the past, all older artificial pacemakers were designed to set the pacing rate (and only one rate) to stimulate the heart, regardless of the patient's needs and the heart's functions. At present, however, almost all newer pacemakers are manufactured as demand pacemakers (it functions only when needed). In addition, most pacemakers are "rate-adaptive." That means that they can be programmed to adjust the pacing rate to your activity level, mimicking your natural heart rhythm. The newer models can meet different pacing needs, depending on where the pacing leads are directed and the method of programming the pulse generator (computer).

Artificial pacemakers can be programmed to adjust the pacing rate to your activity level, mimicking your natural heart rhythm.

In atrioventricular (AV) sequential pacing, the atria (upper chambers) and the ventricles (lower chambers) of your heart are paced sequentially, as the name of the pacing method indicates. In AV sequential pacing, the location of the pacemaker leads allows them to sense your heart's activity and pace as needed: first in the atria and then in the ventricles, sequentially.

Dual-site atrial pacing is still in research. In this type of pacing, the pacemaker programs the leads to stimulate both the right and left atria (both upper chambers). This type of artificial pacing may reduce episodes of atrial fibrillation (an irregular and usually rapid heart rhythm arising from upper chambers; see Question 57).

Biventricular artificial pacing stimulates both the right and left ventricles of your heart. Medical researchers consider this pacing method to be beneficial in improving the pumping action of the heart in patients with advanced congestive heart failure (see Questions 54 and 59).

Currently, all implantable defibrillators (used to shock a heart back into normal rhythm after sudden cardiac arrest or ventricular fibrillation) include artificial pacemaker functions.

Surgery for artificial pacemaker implantation usually requires no more than an overnight hospital stay. In most cases, local anesthesia is used. Before you're discharged from the hospital, doctors program your artificial pacemaker to fit your heart's needs. You would return after several months to allow your doctor to make more detailed adjustments to the pacemaker settings.

82. What are the limits and risks of artificial pacemaker functions?

If you receive an artificial pacemaker implantation, you should carry a wallet ID card showing information about your pacemaker. That's because some equipment used by doctors and dentists can affect your artificial pacemaker functions and may cause it to malfunction. You will also need to show this card when traveling through airports, as the security equipment used to screen passengers should not be used on people with pacemakers.

Many surroundings and devices do not interfere with the function of your artificial pacemaker. They include CB radios, electric drills, electric shavers, electric blankets, heating pads, metal detectors, microwave ovens, TV transmitters, remote control TV changers, and cellular phones (less than 3 watts). Dental equipment does not appear to interfere with the pacemaker functions, but you might may feel an increase in pacing rates during dental drilling.

Electrical shock treatment (electroconvulsive therapy) for certain mental disorders does not appear to interfere with pacemaker functions. Likewise, diagnostic radiation (e.g., chest x ray) appears to show no interference in pacing functions. However, therapeutic radiation (e.g., treatment for certain cancers) may interfere with pacemaker circuits.

Magnetic resonance imaging (MRI) may interfere with your pacemaker functions. Therefore, you should discuss possible risks and benefits with your doctor before undergoing an MRI procedure. Research has shown, however, that **radiofrequency** (RF) **ablation** is safe for pacemaker function. RF is a special electrical treatment to manage a variety of arrhythmias (abnormal heart rhythms; Question 57).

Radiofrequency (RF) ablation

special electrical treatment to manage a variety of rapid heart rhythms.

Lithotripsy

noninvasive treatment to destroy kidney stones.

Performance of **lithotripsy**, a noninvasive treatment to destroy kidney stones, is safe for most pacemaker wearers. However, this treatment may interfere with certain kinds of pacemakers implanted in the abdomen. Also, transcutaneous electrical nerve stimulation to manage acute or chronic pain may interfere with pacemaker function in certain models.

By and large, you should discuss the safety of and possible interference with your pacemaker's functions with physicians or dentists before the use of any medical device or equipment. Pacemaker implantation is a simple procedure involving little risk, and complications are rare. Nevertheless, possible risks and complications do exist.

For example, displacement of the pulse generator or the pacemaker wires (insulated leads) can cause problems. Such events as tearing or perforation of the vein or arterial wall or of your heart itself; puncture of the lungs, which would cause your lung to collapse; and blood clotting or air bubbles in your veins could lead to major medical problems. Other events that would affect your pacemaker include infection or nerve damage at the incision site, bleeding or severe bruising, or even malfunction of your artificial pacemaker itself.

83. What kind of care is necessary after a pacemaker implantation?

After having an artificial pacemaker implanted, every patient requires certain follow-up care. By and large, you can carry out all daily activities without limitation, but you should be familiar with your pacemaker. You need to understand certain precautions and possible risks after receiving a pacemaker.

You should carry a pacemaker ID card at all times; it should contain important information regarding your pacemaker. You would show your ID card to any doctor or dentist or other medical professional during each visit. It's also a good idea to show the ID card to security personnel (e.g., in airports) as needed.

You should discuss the safety of and possible interference with your pacemaker's functions with physicians or dentists.

Treating a Heart Attack

Medical personnel can monitor your pacemaker's functions and transmit them via the telephone using a special telephone transmitter. They connect the transmitter to wristbands on each of your arms, then place the telephone receiver on the transmitter and hold a special magnet over the pacemaker. A specially trained technician on the other end of the phone line checks your heart rate, heart rhythm, pacemaker battery level, and pacemaker functions. The pacemaker check-up via telephone transmitter can be carried out at the doctor's office or at a pacemaker clinic.

You should visit your doctor or a pacemaker clinic several times a year.

Several times a year, you should have a medical check-up at your doctor's office or at a pacemaker clinic. Almost all university or teaching hospitals have a special pacemaker clinic that specializes only in patients with permanent pacemakers. During each visit, technicians check the battery level and functions of your pacemaker and can adjust your pacemaker's settings as needed. The pacemaker pulse generator should be replaced every 6 to 10 years, and the leads may have to be replaced occasionally. The pacemaker clinic also can perform the pacemaker check-up via a telephone transmitter.

Inform your physician immediately if any troubling symptoms or signs occur.

You should take certain precautions after receiving your pacemaker. You must inform your physician immediately if any troubling symptoms or signs occur. For instance, you might notice the reappearance of symptoms that surfaced before your pacemaker was implanted. Or you might feel dizziness, near-syncope or syncope, shortness of breath, marked weakness, or any other symptoms related to heart disease. Additionally, you might develop fever or chills (or both), a very rapid or very slow heart rhythm (with or without palpitations), pain, infection, swelling, or bleeding in the area around your pacemaker, or a swelling of the arm near the incision site. It is vitally important to report any such irregularity at once.

84. What is electrical shock treatment, and who needs it?

There are several ways to manage a variety of cardiac arrhythmias (usually very rapid heart rhythms; see Question 57) with electrical energy. One such process is emergency electrical shock treatment (use of a defibrillator) for cardiac arrest due to ventricular fibrillation (very rapid, chaotic, and ineffective heart rhythm arising from the ventricles; see Question 66). Another is electrical shock treatment of rapid heart rhythms that don't respond to drugs, such as atrial fibrillation (rapid and irregular heart rhythm arising from the upper chambers; see Question 62). Other devices are automatic external defibrillators (AEDs, discussed in Question 85) and implantable cardioverter-defibrillators (ICDs, discussed in Question 86).

Certain drug-resistant rapid heart rhythms require the use of catheter ablation (a nonsurgical technique that destroys parts of the abnormal conduction pathway causing the arrhythmia; see Question 89).

Emergency defibrillation is only a life-saving measure to treat ventricular fibrillation, and the electrical shock should be delivered within 4 minutes from the onset of arrest (ventricular fibrillation). If administered after that, it usually will not prevent a fatal outcome. Delay of shock treatment for more than 4 to 5 minutes often produces permanent brain damage, even if the heart rhythm returns to normal later.

Termination of ventricular tachycardia (very rapid and regular rhythm arising from the lower chambers; see Question 65) also often requires emergency electrical shock treatment. This is especially true if medications are not effective and the arrhythmia is life-threatening. Treatment of cardiac arrest in heart attack victims (see Question 35) usually calls for cardiopulmonary resuscitation (CPR) coupled with electrical shock treatment.

85. What is an automatic external defibrillator, and who needs it?

Patient comment:

If you are considered to be a high-risk patient after recovering from a heart attack, it is an excellent idea to keep an automatic external defibrillator (AED) in your home, especially when you had suffered from several episodes of cardiac arrest in the past. The AED is relatively easy to learn how to operate for anybody, and the device is not too expensive.

Automatic external defibrillator (AED)

portable defibrillator that can deliver an electrical shock to stop ventricular fibrillation.

An **automatic external defibrillator** (AED) is a portable defibrillator that can deliver an electrical shock to halt ventricular fibrillation (very rapid, chaotic, and ineffective heart rhythm arising from the lower heart chambers, discussed in Question 66). The AED is a small portable defibrillator that any lay person can easily operate. It's used before you reach the hospital emergency room (ER). Because ventricular fibrillation must be stopped within a few minutes, an AED can prevent sudden death if used immediately.

Most ambulance teams carry an AED, as do many police and fire rescue units. In addition, AEDs are available in reputable commercial airplanes and various public places, such as sports arenas, large music halls, large international airports, and convention auditoriums. In addition, keeping an AED is highly recommended in private homes for high-risk patients recovering from recent heart attacks. High risks would be seen in those who have had multiple heart attacks, blockage of many coronary arteries, cardiac arrest (ventricular fibrillation), or massive heart muscle damage. Such risks also would include the likelihood of future heart attack, cardiac arrest, or a history of serious complications (see Part 3).

Keeping an AED is highly recommended in private homes for high-risk patients recovering from recent heart attacks.

86. What is an implantable cardioverter-defibrillator, and who needs it?

Recently, the use of implantable cardioverter-defibrillators (ICDs) has been increasingly popular among high-risk heart attack victims. Such a device can prevent sudden death from ventricular fibrillation (see Question 66).

The ICD is a small electronic device that can deliver an electrical shock automatically when you develop ventricular fibrillation or ventricular tachycardia (rapid and regular rhythm arising from the ventricles, as discussed in Question 65). New ICDs provide overdrive pacing to convert sustained ventricular tachycardia and backup pacing for very slow heart rhythm (bradyarrhythmia; see Question 56). The ICDs also provide various other sophisticated functions: noninvasive electrophysiologic (EP) testing and storage of detected arrhythmias (see Question 60).

An ICD consists of two main parts: a pulse generator and leads. The pulse generator is a small lightweight metal case (about the size of a pager or a small match box) containing a small computer and a battery. A surgeon implants the pulse generator under the skin near your left collarbone, usually under general anesthesia. (Some medical centers use local anesthesia and use general anesthesia for shock testing.) The leads are insulated, flexible wires placed in your heart, and they carry electrical energy from the pulse generator to your heart. The surgeon threads most leads from the ICD through one of your veins to the inside of your heart.

The surgery to implant the ICD takes about 2 to 3 hours. Most patients stay in the hospital for 1 to 2 days after the surgery. The cardiologist carries out an electrophysiologic study (EPS) before discharging you to check the device and to evaluate how your ICD is functioning. The cardiologist usually performs a post-surgery EPS and subsequent studies noninvasively through the device via radio waves.

The cardiac team programs and designs each ICD specifically for individual need by performing an EPS before, during, and after the ICD surgery. In that way, your device can retain specific and individualized instructions about your needs. Programming of an ICD uses radio waves, and adjustment of the device can be made externally. An ICD monitors the electrical activity of your heart continuously on a beat-to-beat basis, and it can effectively terminate ventricular fibrillation or tachycardia within seconds.

About 400,000 deaths occur each year in America from sudden cardiac arrest caused by ventricular fibrillation. Most patients who experience this are high-risk heart attack victims. High risk in heart attack victims has been identified previously in Question 85 (see the discussion of automatic external defibrillators). In particular, heart attack victims who survived cardiac arrest belong in the high-risk category. As has been stated, all patients with multiple heart attacks, blockage of multiple arteries, massive heart muscle damage, and major complications are at high risk.

87. What will I feel after an ICD implantation, and what should I do if I receive an electrical shock?

After your ICD implantation, like most patients you will experience some pain and stiffness around the incision area; it may remain swollen and tender for a few weeks. Your surgeon will prescribe some pain medications, but you should avoid any pain medication containing aspirin. If you respond like most patients, you will be discharged from the hospital 1 to 2 days after the surgery. Then you should receive full instructions regarding the functions of your ICD, care of the incision area, physical activity, medications, and various precautions and follow-up visits. Before you are discharged, you will be given an ICD identification card. It contains all necessary information about your ICD: Instructions in case of an emergency, your doctor's name and phone number, and so forth. You should carry this card at all times.

A range of feeling is possible when your ICD is working for rapid heart rhythms. If you developed a rapid heart rhythm, the leads immediately would transmit signals to your ICD to initiate the electrical shock treatment. If the rapid heart rhythm were mild and short in duration, short and rapid electrical pulses would be delivered in a predetermined (programmed) pattern to restore your normal heart rhythm. Such electrical pulses are mild and, like most patients, you wouldn't feel them.

If a very fast abnormal heart rhythm continued, however, your ICD would deliver a much larger electrical shock to terminate the rapid rhythm. Large electrical shocks will be painful, but the discomfort lasts only a fraction of a second. The discomfort is often described as a "kick in the chest."

A large shock is often described as a "kick in the chest."

If you receive an electrical shock, you should sit down or lie down in whatever position you feel more comfortable. A family member or a friend should stay with you throughout the incident. If you were found unconscious, a family member or a friend should call an ambulance (dial 911) and your physician. If the electrical shock seems to be ineffective and the rapid heart rhythm continues, someone should inform your doctor immediately. Dialing 911 might be necessary if you needed any urgent treatment. If your ICD seems to be working properly in response to a rapid heart rhythm, calling your physician immediately isn't necessary.

Your ICD will record and save all necessary information regarding the electrical shock therapy events. The information retrieved from the ICD is very important in evaluating your clinical conditions, the nature of your abnormal heart rhythms, and the effectiveness of your ICD. Thus, medical staff can adjust or reprogram your ICD if necessary to improve its effectiveness.

88. What follow-up care and precautions should I take after I have an ICD implantation?

You should have close communication with your private physician after your ICD is implanted. Before being discharged from the hospital with your ICD, you will receive specific instructions on when to call your physician (or specially trained cardiac nurse). Such instructions would specify calling within 24 hours of receiving an electrical shock; after two or more electrical shocks are received back to back; or if you felt any serious symptoms (e.g., dizziness, near-syncope) from rapid heart rhythm lasting longer than 2 to 3 minutes.

Additionally, your instructions would tell you to call before scheduling any surgical or dental procedures and before scheduling any travel or moving to another location. Naturally, you would call if you had any questions regarding your ICD, medications, or physical activities.

Additional precautions to follow during the first few weeks after your ICD implantation are to avoid lifting anything heavier than 5 to 10 pounds, vigorous exercise or contact sports, and pushing, pulling, or twisting motions and to limit arm movements that may affect the electrical lead (wire) system. Also, you should keep cellular phones at least 6 inches away from your ICD and stay away from magnetic fields, such as high-voltage or strong electrical currents. You should avoid wearing any tight clothing that may irritate the skin over your pulse generator. You should inform your physician of any signs of infection at the incision site or fever above 100°F. Finally, if any medical or dental care is needed, you should inform all medical and dental staff involved regarding your ICD.

Implantation of your ICD requires periodic medical checkups to make certain that the ICD has been effective in halting all rapid heart rhythms. You should schedule follow-up visits several times a year at your doctor's office or at a specially designed clinic dealing with ICDs. During such follow-up visits, medical personnel would use a programmer to guarantee that your ICD detects and treats rapid heart rhythms properly. The programmer also can retrieve various medical information stored in the memory of your ICD.

The medical information includes the events of any rapid heart rhythms to compare with your symptoms and your ICD's effectiveness in handling such events. Your ICD might need reprogramming according to changes in your medical condition and the effectiveness of the device for any rapid heart rhythms, particularly for life-threatening arrhythmias.

You need to replace your ICD's battery every 5 to 8 years as well as the entire generator because its battery is sealed inside. Its battery life depends on the number of electrical shocks and the electrical energy used for stopping rapid heart rhythms. You should have the medical staff test the electrical leads and replace them as needed.

Resuming your daily activities should be gradual, according to your medical condition and your physician's specific instructions. You should avoid driving a car for at least 6 months after being discharged from the hospital. The reason for this is the risk of ventricular arrhythmias (rapid heart rhythms from the lower chambers, discussed in Questions 65 and 66) and not the risk of a problem in the ICD itself. Many patients who experience ventricular arrhythmias may need to avoid driving even after 6 months. Remember that you may develop dizziness, near-syncope, or syncope when ventricular arrhythmias occur. When you experience serious symptoms, you should have your physician evaluate you immediately, and your ICD may need reprogramming.

The natural increase in heart rate during sexual activity should not cause the ICD to deliver an electrical shock. If the ICD delivers an electrical shock during sexual activity, however, you should inform your physician immediately, because your ICD may need reprogramming.

If you schedule any travel, you should consult your physicians beforehand for proper instructions. You should request the name of a cardiologist and hospital in the area (other states or countries) to which you plan to travel. You are highly urged to carry a copy of medical records whenever you schedule an extended trip (longer than 1 month).

You should resume daily activities gradually. They may include walking, swimming, bicycling, bowling, gardening, cooking, golf, tennis, and returning to your previous job (desk job). You should refrain from such sports for the first 4 weeks, however, and any physical activity or emotional stress that may cause a very rapid heart rhythm. Needless to say, you should avoid vigorous or competitive sports and contact sports.

Lots of domestic appliances and devices create no interference with your ICD:

- Televisions, remote controls, tape recorders, radios, garage openers
- Kitchen appliances (toasters, blenders, electric can openers, microwave ovens, electric stoves, refrigerators)
- Washing appliances (electric washers and dryers)

- Sleeping appliances (electric blankets, heating pads)
- Cosmetic appliances (hair dryers, electric shavers)
- Gardening appliances (lawn mowers, leaf blowers)
- Personal computers, printers, fax machines, electric typewriters, copying machines
- Machine shop tools (electric drills, table saws)

Certain other environments, activities, and equipment and devices can cause problems for your ICD:

- MRI (magnetic resonance imaging), radiotherapy, lithotripsy, electrosurgery
- Magnetic fields (high voltage, strong electrical currents, large mechanical or industrial equipment)
- Strong magnets
- Large stereo speakers
- Battery-powered cordless power tools (screwdrivers and drills)
- Leaning over an uncovered running automobile engine
- Malfunctioning electrical or gas-powered appliances
- Being too close (closer than 6 inches) to a cellular phone. (Holding the phone to the ear opposite your implanted side is advisable.)

Your ICD identification card should be shown to airport security personnel because your ICD may set off airport security alarms. Most handheld metal detectors contain a magnet that may interfere with your ICD's functions. Therefore, you should ask security personnel to limit scanning with such devices to less than 30 seconds over the site of the ICD or ask them to search you by hand if possible. At department store and library entrances, you may walk through most theft-detection systems without harm.

89. *What is catheter ablation, and who needs it?*

Catheter ablation (or radio frequency ablation) is a nonsurgical treatment for many kinds of cardiac arrhythmias (abnormal heart rhythms) that are difficult to manage with various medications and other methods. When catheter ablation successfully corrects certain arrhythmias, the procedure is a permanent cure of a given arrhythmia.

The catheter ablation procedure will destroy parts of the abnormal electrical pathway (activity) causing a specific arrhythmia permanently. Thus, catheter ablation in many cases is effective for treating various types of rapid heart rhythms. During catheter ablation, doctors insert under mild local anesthesia a specially designed electrode catheter (a long, thin, flexible tube) into your heart via a vein in your groin or arm. Then they position the catheter in the area of the heart that's causing a specific arrhythmia seen on an x-ray image. At the spot they determine is responsible for the arrhythmia, the electrodes at the tip of the catheter emit radiofrequency energy to destroy the small area of the heart tissue causing the arrhythmia.

Catheter ablation is usually performed in conjunction with an electrophysiologic study (EPS, discussed in Question 60), and the procedure is extremely effective for certain arrhythmias when performed by well-trained cardiac medical teams at well-equipped hospitals. The procedure causes little or no discomfort and has a low risk of complications.

However, since catheter ablation is an invasive procedure that requires the insertion of catheters into the heart, it does carry some small risks with some complications. You may develop bleeding at the insertion site, which could cause local swelling or bruising in the groin or arm. Some rare (but more serious) complications may include damage to your heart tissues and blood vessels, blood clot formation, and infection. If the procedure damages a normal electrical conduction system, you might need an artificial pacemaker.

For a few weeks after catheter ablation, you may experience occasional "skipped" heartbeats and palpitations. Although these symptoms are common, they are benign and self-limited events that will gradually disappear by themselves. However, you should inform your physician immediately if the rapid heart rhythm recurs or if some cardiac symptoms (chest pain, dizziness, shortness of breath, syncope or near-syncope) occur.

Like most patients, you would stay in the hospital overnight after the procedure and be able to resume your usual activities a few days after your discharge from the hospital. When catheter ablation is successful, the procedure will provide a permanent cure for many types of arrhythmias. Thus, the procedure can entirely eliminate a lifetime of many anti-arrhythmic agents (medications to treat various abnormal heart rhythms), leading to a healthy normal life.

PART FIVE

Living After a Heart Attack

What is cardiopulmonary resuscitation, and who needs it?

How much will my attitude contribute to my recovery?

Do I face lifelong medications and check-ups after recovering from a heart attack?

How do I prevent another heart attack?

More ...

90. What is cardiopulmonary resuscitation, and when is it used?

Patient comment:

Everyone should learn how to perform cardiopulmonary resuscitation (CPR), but it's particularly important for family members who live with a heart attack victim. CPR is relatively easy to learn how to perform, and the CPR course is given by many local medical associations and hospitals.

Cardiopulmonary resuscitation (CPR) is urgently necessary when your cardiopulmonary system suddenly and unexpectedly fails to provide adequate and effective function. The purpose of CPR is to restore normal functions of the heart and lungs so that the delivery of adequate oxygen to vital organs—including the heart itself and the brain—is reestablished and maintained. Cardiac arrest most commonly occurs during the first few hours of a heart attack. Remember that permanent brain damage is a common end result when CPR is not applied within 4 minutes, even if cardiac function is restored later. In most cases, cardiac arrest and pulmonary arrest occur together, leading to cardiopulmonary arrest.

Those finding a presumed heart attack victim unconscious as a result of cardiac arrest should immediately seek emergency medical help (dialing 911) and should apply CPR as soon as possible. **A rescuer should not begin CPR until he or she has made sure that the victim is a) not breathing and b) has no heartbeat. CPR performed on a person whose heart is beating can be harmful.** The emergency line operator can give simple instructions over the phone on how to perform

CPR, if no one seems to know the technique, until an ambulance arrives. As described earlier, the most common cause of cardiac arrest is ventricular fibrillation (see Question 66); hence, the use of an automatic external defibrillator (AED), if available, is a life-saving measure if used with performing CPR.

All medical and paramedical personnel must be fully capable of performing CPR. It is highly advisable for the general public to learn the proper technique for CPR because cardiovascular collapse is usually unpredictable. Family members of heart attack victims more urgently need a full understanding of CPR because cardiac patients have a much greater chance of developing cardiac arrest than do healthy people. The technique for CPR is relatively easy to learn, and the local Heart Association and many other medical organizations frequently give CPR courses.

Most hospitals in America commonly use the term **code blue** to designate cardiopulmonary arrest. A CPR team (consisting of specially trained physicians, nurses, and paramedical personnel) is on duty for immediate response to the code blue alert.

Cardiopulmonary arrest causes the loss of certain otherwise observable functions: consciousness (comatose state); pulse (no heartbeat); respiration (no breathing); heart tones (no heart sounds); and blood pressure (BP).

How CPR Is Performed

This rough guide to performing CPR should in no way take the place of CPR instruction. If you wish to be able to perform CPR, you should take a class from

Before you do anything else to help an apparent heart attack victim, call for help!

a certified instructor. However, the description below should provide you with a good idea of what is done in CPR and why it is done. **Before you do anything else to help an apparent heart attack victim, call for help!** Your efforts may be in vain if you do not get the victim to a hospital quickly. CPR is a stop-gap measure only and is no replacement for prompt medical care. Your phone call to 911 is more likely to save the victim than any other action you take.

As stated, the purpose of the initial measure in CPR is to start and maintain the passage of air to the lungs so that adequate amounts of oxygenated blood can be delivered to all organs. Thus, the initial measure should follow the ABC guide: clearing the Airway (the route by which air travels to the lungs), starting and maintaining Breathing, and restoring blood Circulation.

As noted above, it is important to begin by making sure that the victim is incapable of breathing on his or her own, and to check for a heartbeat. In some cases, the victim may not be breathing, but still have heart activity—often ventricular fibrillation (VF), which is commonly associated with heart attacks. If VF is evident, those administering CPR should deliver a forceful blow to the sternum (around the breastbone) with the heel of the hand; they may repeat the blow once or twice more if that produces no response. A direct blow to the sternum can terminate VF and may restore normal heart rhythm. If this maneuver is not successful, however, help should immediately proceed to the next step.

Airway

The first maneuver in CPR should be to place the patient in a supine (lying down, face-up) position. The person performing CPR should place one hand behind

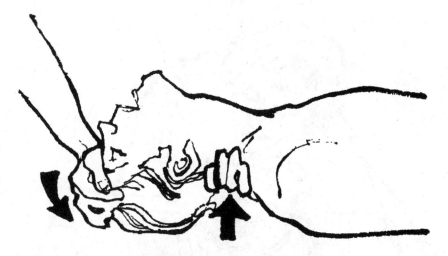

Figure 11   CPR step 1: tilt the head back to open the airway.

the patient's neck and the other hand on the forehead (Figure 11). When the head is tilted back, this maneuver lifts the tongue from the back of the throat so that the patient's airway will be fully open. During this maneuver, the rescuer should remove any obvious foreign body in the mouth and airway. For many patients, this maneuver alone may be enough to restore breathing and to start recovery from cardiovascular arrest. The person providing CPR should put his or her ear over the mouth to listen for breath sounds. If the victim is breathing, no further direct action is required unless the breathing stops, but the victim should be continually monitored and transported to a hospital in an ambulance as soon as possible.

Breathing

If the victim is not breathing, CPR providers should maintain the backward tilt of the patient's head with one hand and pinch the nostrils closed with the other hand. The rescuer should place his or her mouth over the patient's mouth, completely sealing it to avoid any

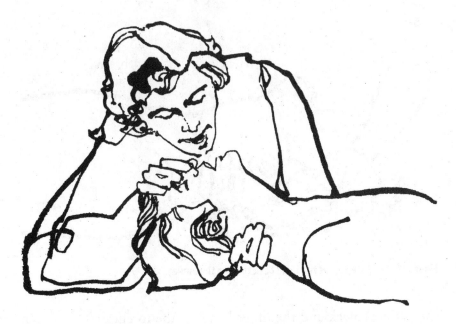

Figure 12   CPR step 2: if the patient can't breathe on his own, begin artificial respiration.

leak of air (Figure 12). At the end of inspiration (breathing in), one should exhale (blow out) a longer-than-usual breath into the patient's mouth. Artificial (mouth-to-mouth) respiration should be performed at a rate of 12 breaths per minute. If the technique is correct, a rise should be noted in the patient's chest. If the chest does not rise, the rescuer should check again for blockages in the airway, make sure the nose is pinched, and readjust the mouth position to prevent leakage. There should be no loss of air through the nose or mouth as the lungs inflate. After inflation of the lungs, one should remove the mouth from the patient's mouth, allowing the patient's lungs to deflate. Air should be heard escaping from the lungs during that period. A pause of about five seconds should be enough to allow the lungs to deflate before the next breath.

The principle of mouth-to-nose resuscitation is essentially the same as that of mouth-to-mouth resuscitation. In this technique, while maintaining the backward tilt with one hand, the CPR provider should close the patient's jaw and seal the patient's mouth with the other hand. Then, one would place the mouth over the patient's nose and, after inhaling deeply, would exhale into the patient's nose. Artificial respiration should be performed at a rate of 12 breaths per minute.

Circulation

If the patient is not breathing and has no heartbeat (determined by feeling for a pulse in the neck or groin for about 5 seconds), the next step in the initial resuscitation measures is the application of cardiac massage. Closed-chest cardiac massage is recommended in practically all clinical circumstances except when the patient is already in the operating room or when chest wounds don't allow closed-chest massage.

To perform cardiac massage, the patient's back must be placed on a firm surface. When the patient is on a soft surface (e.g., a bed), a hard board should be placed under the back. The reason for this is that you cannot compress the heart to pump blood adequately if the surface is soft under the victim. While standing alongside the patient, the rescuer places the heel of one hand over the lower third of the patient's sternum; a common rule of thumb is to find the tip of the breastbone where the ribs meet and place your hand three fingers' width up from that point. Only the heel of the hand should be in touch with the patient's chest. The other hand may rest on the first hand (Figure 13).

The rescuer then compresses the patient's chest 1.5 to 2 inches; the pressure should be smooth and uninterrupted. After that compression, the rescuer must release the sternum and ready the hand for the next

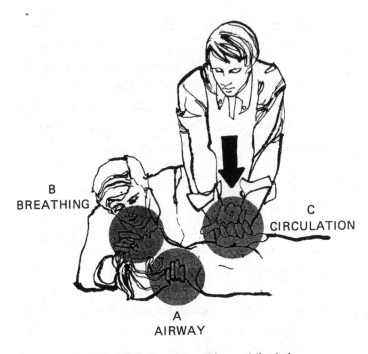

B
BREATHING

C
CIRCULATION

A
AIRWAY

Figure 13   The ABCs of CPR: Airway, Breathing, and Circulation.

compression. The duration of the chest compression should be similar to that of relaxation; that is, the amount of time spent doing the compression equals the time spent between compressions. The chest should be compressed about 60 times per minute and coordinated with artificial respiration. If only one person is present, 15 chest compressions are recommended, followed by two quick artificial respirations. When two or more persons are available for CPR, every fifth chest compression should be followed by one lung ventilation (artificial respiration). To check the success of closed-chest cardiac massage, **peripheral pulses** (e.g., pulses on the neck or groin area) should be felt periodically—every minute or so—because, as stated above, if the rescuer is successful in restoring a heartbeat, the compressions should be halted.

Peripheral pulse

pulse in the arms or legs.

During the initial measures of CPR, one must check for several signs that indicate the success or failure of the resuscitative efforts. Important signs include pulse in the arm, groin, or neck arteries; heart tones (sounds); spontaneous breathing; and palpable or recordable BP. Of course, one should also be alert to any change in the patient's neurologic status and in the status of consciousness.

When there is any evidence that resuscitative efforts have been successful, the rescuer may stop and observe the patient for several seconds. If the cardiovascular collapse has stopped, one should continue to observe the patient very closely. When resuscitative efforts have been successful outside a hospital setting, ambulance personnel should transport the patient promptly to a nearby ER. Needless to say, paramedic personnel of the ambulance will take over the CPR efforts as soon as they arrive at the scene. If, however, there is no change in the patient's status, those in attendance must continue artificial respiration and cardiac massage (Figures 12 and 13) until an ambulance arrives. They should not stop CPR for longer than 5 seconds.

After CPR

Various complications of closed-chest cardiac massage may occur, although the procedure is relatively safe in most instances. When treating children and elderly people, one must not be overly vigorous in chest compression to avoid any unnecessary damage to the ribs, sternum, and various organs. Complications of cardiac massage may include fracture of the ribs and sternum; **hemothorax** (bleeding in the chest cavity); **hemopericarium** (bleeding in the sac surrounding the heart); pneumothorax (collapse of the lungs); rupture of the

Living After a Heart Attack

Hemothorax

accumulation or blood in the chest cavity.

Hemopericardium

accumulation of blood in pericardial sac.

stomach or the aorta (the largest arterial trunk); laceration of the liver and spleen; and bone marrow embolism (blood clots in the bone marrow; see Question 38).

After successful CPR, assessment of the underlying cause of the cardiopulmonary arrest is essential. Thus, the cardiac care unit (CCU) staff should closely observe and treat any patient who has recovered from cardiopulmonary arrest. First, they must manage the underlying heart disease (e.g., heart attack; see Question 68) together with the major complications (e.g., life-threatening arrhythmias, CHF, and the like; see Question 59). Some patients may require an implantable cardioverter-defibrillator (ICD; see Question 86), an artificial pacemaker (see Question 80), or various medications, depending upon the clinical circumstance. Of course, the treatment of the underlying heart disease—heart attack—is essential. Thus, some patients may need coronary angioplasty (see Question 72) or coronary artery bypass graft (see Question 77). It should be noted that after a massive heart attack, some patients may develop cardiopulmonary arrest again after recovery from their first arrest. Therefore, medical staff must monitor even more closely any heart attack victim with extensive heart muscle damage or multiple artery blockage.

Feature

Conversation with a Patient Recovered from a Heart Attack

Mr. Benjamin Han is a 67-year-old retired banker (vice-president of one of the major banks) who had suffered from a heart attack 13 to 14 years ago and recovered from a heart attack without any complication. Coronary angioplasty was performed with a stent. His coronary risk factors included diabetes mellitus, abnormal blood cholesterol levels, occasional smoking, type-A personality, and some stress (job-related). His wife is a retired dentist. The following questions and answers are a candid conversation with the patient.

Q. What was the first symptom you experienced upon the onset of your heart attack?

A. On day 1, I experienced a short but severe pain in my left chest, and the pain was sharp enough to stop my routine daily walk outside of my office. I did not take it seriously at that time, but, in retrospect, it must have been a warning sign of the oncoming heart attack the next day.

Q. Did you feel any type of chest discomfort, significant shortness of breath, tingling sensation or numbness in the arms or shoulders?

A. Soon after lunch on day 2 on the way back to my office, I felt my breathing was short, uneven, and uncomfortable. My face was pale enough for co-workers to notice. My feeling then was that I must be having a not-so-unusual indigestion problem.

Q. Did you experience marked weakness, dizziness, or feeling of a fainting spell?

A. My pale face coincided with a sense of dizziness. I do not remember actual syncope, but I remember that I was not in a talking mood, as I felt weak and uncomfortable.

Q. What were you doing when you experienced any of the above-mentioned symptoms?

A. I was waiting in front of an elevator after walking back from my lunch. My walk was not at a routine pace, however.

Q. What action did you first take when you considered that you might be having a possible heart attack?

A. As I was returning to my office, my secretary first noticed my pale face and she commented on it. As she realized my weakness and my reluctance to converse with her, her friend who happened to be visiting her remarked that I must be having a heart attack. Her friend, I found out later, was a former nurse. Her suggestion was to go to the hospital. I hesitated initially, disbelieving what I heard. However, my secretary insisted on calling my personal friend, the cardiologist Dr. Edward Chung at Thomas Jefferson University Hospital, and I finally called Dr. Chung reluctantly.

Q. How soon did you go to a nearby hospital emergency room (ER)?

A. Upon hearing my medical history over the phone, Dr. Chung considered strongly that I was having a heart attack, and he ordered me to call an ambulance and come to his hospital ER right away.

Q. What mediations were given to you in the ER and what diagnostic tests were performed?

A. I believe that I was given a thrombolytic agent (later found out that it was tPA—tissue plasminogen activator), and a series of blood tests with an ECG was performed.

Q. *What additional diagnostic tests and treatment were performed when you were transferred to the CCU?*

A. Cardiac catheterization with coronary angiogram (arteriogram) before performing coronary angioplasty.

Q. *Was coronary angioplasty performed? How many blood vessels (arteries) were dilated?*

A. My team of doctors performed coronary angioplasty on my left anterior descending artery. I had a second angioplasty on the same coronary artery with a stent implantation 6 months later because of restenosis. At that time, the use of a stent was somewhat experimental and not yet widely used.

Q. *Was coronary artery bypass graft performed? How many blood vessels were treated?*

A. No bypass surgery was performed.

Q. *Did you suffer from any significant complications such as congestive heart failure and abnormal heart rhythms?*

A. Fortunately, I did not have any complications.

Q. *Did you experience angina (chest discomfort) or any other cardiac symptoms prior to this heart attack?*

A. I might have experienced a sense of sluggishness and weak muscle strength. The briefcase I carried in the morning felt burdensome. But I did not know all these feelings were related to the heart attack. I do not recall any chest discomfort (angina) in the past.

Q. How long did you stay in the hospital?

A. It must have been for about 10 days. Hospital stay at the time was not restrictive.

Q. How many medications are you taking after your discharge from the hospital?

A. Initially, I was taking aspirin and atenol everyday. Later, I added a series of vitamins C, E, and folic acid. Now, I take two baby aspirins a day, folic acid, and Zocor (cholesterol-lowering drug).

Q. Are there significant changes in your lifestyle, diet, physical exercises, and coronary risk factors?

A. My wife has been very conscientious about my diet (e.g., lean meat, balanced healthy foods) Although I preferred high cholesterol foods, I have been listening to my wife's advice 95% of the time. I have switched my regular exercise from tennis to golf, following my doctor's recommendation. I have an exercise routine of walking three times a week and golfing three to four times a week. I have been very deliberate in all my efforts in minimizing stress—trying not be emotionally charged, and avoiding any cause of anxiety, if at all possible.

Q. Do you have any contributing risk factors (coronary risk factors) such as smoking, family history, high blood pressure, diabetes mellitus, high cholesterol, obesity, etc.?

A. Most of my siblings seem to have a history of high cholesterol, but none seem to show high blood pressure. I am the only one in my immediate family who has diabetes, which came to me in my early 50s. I must have had a stressful career and environment. I smoked irregularly and moderately before the heart attack. Since then, I quit smoking completely.

91. How much will my attitude contribute to my recovery? How do I live after having had a heart attack?

After recovering from a heart attack, you have two major goals. One is the development of a special individual plan to restore your emotional as well as your physical ability to return to a normal and healthy life. The second is control of all coronary risk factors to prevent a second heart attack. Thus, cardiac rehabilitation programs focus on three main areas: regular medical check-ups with proper medications, lifestyle adjustment with proper changes, and emotional adjustment.

It is extremely important to remember that the underlying coronary atherosclerotic process (hardening of the coronary arteries) has not disappeared or stopped even if you have been lucky enough to recover from a heart attack. In addition, it should be stressed that a second heart attack is often more serious than the first attack. Thus, recovery from a second heart attack may be even more difficult and your chances lessened. Therefore, in recovery you must control, minimize, or eliminate all coronary risk factors (see Question 16) more carefully to prevent a second heart attack.

Your doctor can help you decide whether cholesterol-lowering medications would be useful. Such medications are recommended in following situations:

- Markedly elevated total cholesterol more than 240 mg/dL and/or markedly elevated LDL (bad) cholesterol more than 160 mg/dL, particularly with low HDL (good) cholesterol less than 35 mg/dL. Cholesterol-lowering medications may be used when low-cholesterol diets and physical exercise aren't effective.

• Moderately abnormal cholesterol levels that are present despite a low-cholesterol diet with proper exercise, especially when one or more additional risk factors are present or coronary artery disease has already been diagnosed.

There are many cholesterol-lowering medications (e.g., Lipitor, Zocor, Mevacor) available for clinical use, but proper medication for each patient will be determined by his or her physician depending upon the clinical circumstances. It is very important to remember that every individual with known coronary risk factors should be evaluated and treated regularly by his or her physician.

92. How do I prevent another heart attack?

Patient comment:

When you are lucky enough to recover from a heart attack, you should try very hard to prevent the second heart attack. As you already know by now, the underlying process of the hardening of arteries (atherosclerosis) that causes a heart attack never stops. Therefore, coronary risk factors must be controlled as best you can.

Your risk of another heart attack can be greatly lowered by using the common-sense approaches listed below.

• **Have regular medical check-ups.** Regular medical check-ups are highly recommended even for apparently healthy people (men above the age of 35 and women above 40) to make certain that any coronary risk factors (see Part 2) or any signs of heart diseases are discovered. Regular medical check-ups should consist of the baseline blood tests, including blood levels of cholesterols and triglycerides, and resting ECG. When any abnormalities show up in the test results or when your doctor detects any abnormal physical findings during a medical check-up, various additional diagnostic tests (e.g., echocardiogram, stress ECG test, coronary angiogram, and **cardiac catheterization**) may be necessary. When any known coronary risk factor, particularly a hereditary factor, is found, regular medical check-ups are needed even for much younger people.

Cardiac catheterization

invasive diagnostic cardiac test that measures pressures in various locations within the heart chambers and blood vessels, and any other cardiac findings.

- **Eliminate or control coronary risk factors.** Millions of people have one or more coronary risk factors, but many people do not know about them or simply ignore them. The hereditary factor is beyond your control, but the remaining coronary risk factors can be controlled if you are motivated enough to understand them and to try hard to reduce their effects. Smoking is just one major coronary risk factor that can be completely eliminated if the individual is willing to work hard to eliminate it from his or her life—and the prospect of another heart attack can provide high motivation. Remember that multiple coronary risk factors have a cumulative effect (that is, they multiply the effects of each individual factor) which speeds up the atherosclerotic process (process of hardening of arteries) so that it can occur very rapidly even among young people.

Remember that there are often few or no symptoms in the presence of various coronary risk factors, such as high BP (hypertension), abnormal blood cholesterol levels, and diabetes—this is why heart disease is called a "silent killer." Thus, there is no way of knowing these risk factors unless regular medical check-ups with the baseline diagnostic tests are performed.

- **Eat a healthy diet.** A healthy diet consists of low-calorie foods with a lot of vegetables, fruits, fish, and chicken (without skin). Consumption of cholesterol-rich foods, such as red meats (e.g., beef, pork), butter, egg yolk, cheese, and ice cream, should be kept to a minimum. The average person should consume approximately 2,000 calories a day for good health.

- **Get regular exercise.** It is highly recommended to engage in a regular and proper exercise program throughout life. Recommended exercise may include brisk walking, jogging, swimming, dancing (moderate tempo), golfing and tennis (not competitive).

This does not mean you must join a gym or work out strenuously for hours on end. You do not need to become a "hard body" to have good health. Even a person who is overweight with high BP, abnormal blood cholesterol levels, and diabetes will see significant benefits from an exercise program of walking 30 minutes a day 3 to 4 times a week. Exercise is also improves emotional well being; a person who follows a simple, regular exercise program will feel happier and less stressed.

A person who follows a simple, regular exercise program will feel happier and less stressed.

- **Avoid overexertion.** For people with heart problems, there are some limitations. You should avoid physical exercise on a very cold or hot day (especially with high humidity). Shoveling a snow-covered driveway on a cold day is extremely dangerous for older people, particularly those with coronary risk factors. Likewise, you should avoid any exercise for 1 to 2 hours after a heavy meal and/or alcohol consumption. Vigorous or competitive sports among older adults, particularly with known coronary risk factors or a previous history of heart attack(s), are rather dangerous and may even be fatal. Playing any sport alone is not advisable for people with coronary risk factors.

- **Limit alcohol consumption.** Alcohol use is not a coronary risk factor, but excessive consumption can be harmful in many ways. Alcohol may trigger various abnormal heart rhythms and may raise BP. In addition, excessive consumption of alcohol causes **cardiomyopathy** (heart muscle disease) and can reduce the pumping action of the heart in people with congestive heart failure (diminished pumping action of the heart). Alcohol may also produce abnormal blood levels of cholesterol and triglyceride.

Cardiomyopathy
heart muscle disease.

- **Avoid stress.** Unnecessary stress should be avoided as much as possible, particularly for older adults and people with coronary risk factors and/or previous heart attack(s). People who habitually experience strong negative emotions, particularly anger, have a much higher likelihood of heart attacks than those who are realistic, optimistic, generous, and happy. It is not unusual for angry people, particularly men, to suffer a heart attack before the age of 40 even without other coronary risk factors. Therefore, practices that help to calm anger and other strong emotion can help prevent heart attacks. Techniques such as meditation, anger management instruction, yoga, tai chi, and exercise can be useful in learning to avoid negative emotions.

Practices that help to calm anger and other strong emotion can help prevent heart attacks.

- **Ask for cooperation and support from your spouse or partner.** If you are in a marriage or long-term relationship, it is extremely important to have full cooperation and support from your partner, particularly for older adults and people with known coronary risk factors or previous heart attack(s). Eating a healthy diet often requires your spouse to change his or her eating and cooking habits as well, so it is crucial that your spouse work with you. As you try to change your lifestyle to reduce your risk of heart attack, pay attention to your relationship with your spouse or partner, and seek ways to reduce the stress of your life changes on both of you.

- **Avoid denial.** Many people have a tendency to deny their symptoms of a heart attack; they hope that if they ignore it, it will go away, or tell themselves that it is "all in my head." As a result, they delay the emergency medical care they need, with potentially serious consequences. Remember that early recognition of symptoms and early medical care often influences the "life and death" outcome. When medical care is delayed, full recovery from a heart attack is difficult to expect, and many major complications (see Part 4) occur—including death, which can potentially be avoided if there are no delays in care. Do not risk your life! If you experience symptoms consistent with heart attacks, seek medical attention. It is better to act and find out you were mistaken about the symptoms than to do nothing and suffer the consequences.

- **Avoid self-diagnosis and self-treatment**. When a patient happens to be a physician, dentist, nurse, paramedic, or someone working in the hospitals or medical research institutions, there is a tendency to make "self diagnosis" followed by providing "self-treatment." This is rather a dangerous and unacceptable way to handle a heart attack, because you do not have control over your physical capabilities

It is better to act and find out you were mistaken about the symptoms than to do nothing and suffer the consequences.

when you're experiencing such a serious medical problem. The temptation to provide your own medical care must be absolutely avoided so that your emergency medical care is not delayed. If you are a health care professional, you would likely advise patients not to try to treat themselves, but to seek help instead—so take your own advice and summon help if you need it.

- **Learn CPR, and encourage others to do so.** All lay people should learn how to perform CPR because unexpected cardiopulmonary arrest can occur at any time. The CPR technique is relatively easy to learn, and the American Heart Association and many other medical organizations provide CPR teaching courses on a regular basis. It is particularly important for family members of heart attack victims or people with multiple coronary risk factors. Obviously, you cannot perform CPR upon yourself, but if everyone in your family (including you) learns to perform CPR, you will be much safer should you have another heart attack.

- **Live near a major hospital.** It is advisable to live in any relatively large city not far (driving distance) from any major hospital with qualified medical staff and well-equipped medical facilities. This is especially important for older adults and people with multiple coronary risk factors and a history of a previous heart attack. By doing so, proper medical care can be provided without delay. If you already live in such a location, that's no problem—but if you do not, you might wish to weigh the possibility of moving to a place within range of a hospital. Whether you make such a move depends on the severity of your heart condition; you should discuss the matter with your doctor before deciding to move or stay. It might seem to be a big transition to make, particularly if your home is in a rural area, but remember that heart disease kills quickly and sometimes without much warning; deciding to move might just be a life and death decision.

- **Take daily aspirin.** Aspirin acts as an anticoagulant and helps prevent blockages in the bloodstream, so it can reduce chances of a heart attack in people with coronary artery disease. Daily intake of aspirin (81 mg) is recommended for most adults unless there are overriding reasons why they should not take it. Aspirin should not be taken by people with recent head trauma, peptic ulcer, recent surgery, or bleeding disorders, for example. Your doctor can tell you whether you have any conditions that might prevent you from safely taking aspirin.

Daily intake of aspirin is recommended for most adults unless there are overriding reasons why they should not take it.

93. Do I face lifelong medications and check-ups after recovering from a heart attack?

For most people, it takes about 2 to 3 months to return to usual (normal) life. Therefore, the first 2 to 3 months after being discharged from the hospital are very important not only for you but for all your family members, particularly your spouse.

It is essential for you to have regular medical check-ups throughout your entire life after recovering from a heart attack. During each visit, your doctor will evaluate your cardiac status, will perform any necessary tests (e.g., blood tests, electrocardiograms, and the like), and may adjust your medications as needed. If necessary, your doctor will perform additional tests, such as a stress test, an echocardiogram, or a coronary angiogram (see

Question 51) depending upon medical evaluation. In addition, your doctor may add new medications and may have to change the dosage of certain medications according to your cardiac status. Evaluation will include various functions of any medical devices (e.g., artificial pacemaker; see Question 80). Your physician should be notified immediately if any new symptom occurs or a preexisting symptom gets worse. Close communication with your physician and regular medical check-ups should be a part of your life's routines.

94. Do heart attack survivors have to continue on medications?

Many patients who recover from a heart attack need one or more medications for a long time (and often for their entire lifetime). Many patients who recover from a heart attack need a variety of medications to control high blood pressure (BP). Doctors usually prescribe antihypertensive medications (see Question 26) for their entire lifetime to those who have high BP, unless their physicians give special instructions to do otherwise.

When your blood cholesterol levels are markedly abnormal and low-cholesterol diets and physical exercise are not effective, you may need a variety of cholesterol-lowering medications under medical supervision (e.g., statins, niacin, and the like).

Medical experts recommend beta-blockers (see Question 69) for every patient for 1 year or more after recovery from a heart attack. These beta-blockers reduce your heart rate and BP to lessen the demands on your heart. In a recent major study, the beta-blocker Coreg® was shown to reduce risk of death among

Living After a Heart Attack

heart attack patients with impaired cardiac function by 23%.

Calcium-channel blockers help to relax the muscles of your blood vessels and often slow your heart rate. Blood-thinning medications (anticoagulants) make blood less sticky, so they can help to prevent blood clot formation. Doctors recommend them highly for most people who recover from a heart attack. A daily aspirin is the ideal medication for this purpose, unless you demonstrate obvious reasons for avoiding them (e.g., recent surgery, peptic ulcer, and the like). For some people, their doctor may prescribe a blood thinner stronger than aspirin.

Some people with clinically significant arrhythmias (abnormal heart rhythms; see Question 57) need one or more medications under close medical supervision to control or to prevent arrhythmias. Thus, you may require antiarrhythmic medications even after implantation of an artificial pacemaker or ICD (see Questions 80 and 86).

If you had a moderate to severe heart attack associated with major complications (congestive heart failure or cardiogenic shock), angiotensin-converting enzyme (ACE) inhibitors (see Question 69) are highly beneficial in improving blood circulation of your coronary arteries and improving the pumping action of your heart.

Many patients who recover from a heart attack may need additional medications. For example, if you were diabetic, you would need insulin or other medication to control your diabetes. Also, you might require other medications depending upon coexisting diseases.

95. *What activities should I avoid after a heart attack?*

Patient comment:

Even though regular physical exercise is extremely beneficial after recovering from a heart attack, you should avoid certain activities. For example, you should avoid any competitive or vigorous sports beyond what your heart can take. Any competitive sport has a tendency to create emotional tension and anxiety that cause unnecessary stress, which is harmful to your heart. The stress may provoke angina or abnormal heart rhythms and may raise your blood pressure. Even betting money during any sport or game is not recommended for anyone who recovered from a heart attack in order to avoid unnecessary stress. The key is: Stay relaxed! Things that make you anxious should be eliminated.

For anyone who recovers from a heart attack, it is absolutely important to stop smoking. As emphasized repeatedly, smoking is a major coronary risk factor that you can eliminate completely (see Question 16). There are methods available to help you quit if you are unable to do so on your own; contact the American Lung Association for information on quitting smoking. Alcohol is not directly harmful if you consume only a small amounts, e.g., one to two glasses of wine with dinner, depending on your tolerance for alcohol; you should not drink a quantity that is likely to get you tipsy or drunk. However, alcohol may trigger some abnormal heart rhythms (see Question 57) and reduce the pumping action of your heart. Thus, you are advised to take alcohol (even small amounts) under close medical supervision.

You should avoid vigorous competitive or contact sports. You should avoid sudden physical exercise, such as rapid dancing, running, or playing singles tennis, soon after meals or alcohol consumption. Any physical activity on very cold or hot days (especially with high humidity) is very dangerous, and you should avoid it. In particular, cleaning a snow-covered driveway on a cold day is extremely dangerous—it is actually almost suicidal for a person recovering from a heart attack to do this.

Driving an automobile is safe only about 3 to 4 weeks after your discharge from the hospital. Doctors recommend initially driving a short distance for half an hour or less. You should avoid rush hour traffic if possible. If you have received an ICD, you may have to wait longer until you can safely drive because of the danger of provoking serious abnormal heart rhythms (see Question 57) during driving. If any cardiac symptoms occur during your driving, you should contact your physician for further recommendation.

You should minimize emotional stress as much as possible after your recovery from a heart attack. Emotional stress causes a fast heart rate, raises your BP, and increases your heart's workload. You should learn how to be realistic and optimistic and to relax. Regular exercise and an optimistic attitude are very important in reducing any stress, and you should try hard to be happy. There are many options—classes, self-help books, etc.—for learning to manage your emotions if you don't know how. If you are a chronically unhappy or angry person, consider counseling with a minister or psychological professional to address long-term emotional problems—it could be a life-or-death effort.

It is very important also for you to maintain a proper healthy diet after recovering from your heart attack, especially if you have abnormal blood cholesterol levels (see Question 17) or are obese. You should markedly minimize your intake of high-cholesterol foods, including red meat from four-legged animals, egg yolk, butter, cheese, certain seafood (shrimp, lobster, crab, clams, oysters), ice-cream, and whole milk (see Questions 20 and 21). You should eat more of a variety of fish (e.g., mackerel and salmon), which contain omega–3 fatty acids, and eat egg white in place of egg yolks. Fruits and vegetables and proper exercise can benefit you considerably.

By and large, if you are overweight, you should not overeat and should markedly reduce your calorie intake. Remember that the risk of coronary heart disease, including heart attack, increases significantly even if you are just 10% overweight. In addition, if you lose just 5 to 10 pounds, you can reduce your BP. If you need to lose weight, talk to your physician or ask for a referral to a nutritionist. Sometimes, weight loss can be best accomplished by educating yourself about what you can and cannot eat, and how much you should eat.

96. Will physical activity help to build up my body after a heart attack?

Proper exercise is beneficial for heart attack survivors. Before engaging in any exercise program, however, you should discuss your exercise plan in advance with your physician. Medical researchers highly recommend performing a stress test (exercise ECG test) to determine your exact ability to engage in any physical activity (see Question 48). By doing so, your doctor can scientifically measure your heart's **functional capacity** (your ability to perform physical activity).

Functional capacity

ability to perform physical activity.

Exercise is proven to be a major component of a cardiac rehabilitation program. Exercise is beneficial in improving the heart muscle function after a heart attack. In addition, the beneficial effects of exercise include maintaining a healthy body weight, blood pressure, and blood cholesterol levels and in controlling diabetes. Regular physical exercise usually reduces emotional stress. The American Heart Association recommends proper healthy physical exercise, such as brisk walking, bicycling, swimming, jogging, and dancing, for 30 minutes at least three to four times a week. Every individual should start any exercise program gradually and not abruptly.

Every individual should start any exercise program gradually.

There is no set time schedule for when to resume a sexual relationship after you recover from a heart attack. However, it is relatively safe to resume sexual activity a few weeks after your discharge from the hospital. Resuming a sexual relationship should be gradual, and you should be certain that you are free of any cardiac symptoms (chest discomfort, shortness of breath, tired feeling, dizziness, and palpitations). You should select any sexual position that requires less physical effort, and you should feel comfortable. If any abovementioned symptom occurs during sexual activity, you should stop immediately and inform your physician. You should avoid sexual activity within 2 hours after meals or alcohol consumption.

Sexual relationships with a much younger person and/or extramarital affairs are not recommended, because overexcitement may be dangerous to you. In considering sexual activity, you should consult your physician first. Some medications may cause unexpected side effects, especially when you are taking several medications together.

Returning to work is a reasonable physical activity provided that you avoid the above-mentioned risks. Most people will be able to return to work about 3 to 4 weeks after discharge from the hospital. Several factors will determine the exact time of your return to work, however: the degree of heart muscle damage, severity of various complications (see Question 59), speed of recovery, and the type of work.

Initially, your return to work should be gradual and progressive, as you can tolerate it. It is a good idea for you to work only half a day at first and gradually increase your work to a full day. If you job is very physically demanding, such as work involving manual labor, you may have to change your occupation to one that demands less physical work (e.g., a desk job).

Initially, your return to work should be gradual.

97. Must I be careful in taking medications for other ailments?

If you have known diseases or disorders such as diabetes mellitus, high blood pressure, abnormal heart rhythms (cardiac arrhythmias) etc., you may need one or more medications for many months, years, or even indefinitely. You should always be careful when you require two or more medications because every drug has a specific pharmacological effect that may increase or decrease the potency of one or more medications. This is true when dealing with any prescription drug or nonprescription drug (even over-the-counter medication).

Even when you need to take a simple, commonly used medication such as antacid or cough medicine from a local drug store, you should consult your physician beforehand because unexpected side effects may occur. Remember that some medications may trigger abnormal heart rhythms, and some other drugs may decrease the pumping action of the heart. These undesirable side effects are harmful to heart attack victims, especially during the first few weeks after recovering from a heart attack.

If you already have or happen to develop stomach ulcer or any bleeding disorder, you should avoid using aspirin or any anticoagulant (blood thinning drug) such as coumadin. Likewise, these medications should not be used during and soon after any major surgery or trauma, or even for a dental procedure. Under these circumstances, you should, or course, consult your physician for proper advice.

98. Is my heart in danger if I undergo surgery for other ailments?

There is no direct effect on your heart when you undergo surgery for other diseases (e.g., surgery for any intestinal problem such as appendectomy). However, the fear or anxiety before any major surgery will produce some stress to your heart, especially soon after recovering from a heart attack. A stressful situation may trigger cardiac arrhythmias (abnormal heart rhythms) or angina (chest pain), and may raise your blood pressure if you already have significant hypertension.

If you need another type of heart surgery, such as a heart valve replacement, after recovering from a heart attack, the damaged heart will obviously receive more stress. Needless to say, you should consult your physician in advance when any surgery is needed. When any major surgery is scheduled, some medications may have to be changed or even stopped temporarily.

99. Are heart attack victims ever pronounced completely cured?

Heart attacks are different from other diseases such as appendicitis or pneumonia. From the viewpoint of its nature and the disease process, it is difficult to say whether the heart attack can be cured completely.

Nevertheless, in a way, it can be said that the heart attack can be cured completely when coronary angioplasty, thrombolytic therapy, or coronary artery bypass graft has been successful without any significant complication, and you become symptom-free.

Remember, however, that the underlying disease process, namely, atherosclerosis (hardening of arteries), will continue in most patients after recovering from a heart attack, especially when various coronary risk factors are *not* well controlled. Thus, from this explanation, we may say that the heart attack can be cured completely, but the disease that led to it, atherosclerosis, *cannot* be cured.

100. Where can I find more information about heart attack?

You may request brochures or various booklets produced by the American Heart Association, American College of Cardiology, pharmaceutical companies, and many teaching hospitals or university hospitals regarding a variety of topics. These include heart attack and related subjects such as high blood pressure, proper exercise and diets, cholesterol, smoking, arrhythmias, stress testing, electrophysiology study, artificial pacemakers, cardiac catheterization, coronary angioplasty, coronary stent, and coronary artery bypass graft. These booklets are available to the general public free of charge from any local medical association or large community and University hospitals.

For further information, you can refer to the Appendix that follows.

Organizations

American Heart Association
American Heart Association National Center
National Center
7272 Greenville Avenue
Dallas, TX 75231
Phone: 800-AHA-US-1 or 1-800-242-8721
Web site: *www.americanheart.org*
Note that you can access information for local chapters of the AHA using your
    local telephone book or clicking on "Your Local AHA Office" in the "Contact
    Us" tab on the AHA web site.

Centers for Disease Control and Prevention
1600 Clifton Rd.
Atlanta, GA 30333
Phone (for public inquiries): (404) 639-3534
(800) 311-3435
Web site: *www.cdc.gov*

National Institutes of Health/National Heart, Lung, and Blood Institute
NHLBI Health Information Center
Attention: Web Site
P.O. Box 30105
Bethesda, MD 20824-0105
Phone: 301 592 8573; (TTY): 240 629 3255
Web site: *www.nhlbi.nih.gov/index.htm*

Heart Health Web Sites

This list is not comprehensive, but the sites here contain many links to other
    valuable sites.

American Heart Association: *www.americanheart.org*
Centers for Disease Control & Prevention: *www.cdc.gov/cvh/*
Early Heart Attack Care: *http://ehac.chestpain.org/st-agnes/splashnews2.html*
Johns Hopkins Hospital:
   www.hopkinsmedicine.org/heartdisease.html
Massachusetts General Hospital Health and Wellness Information: *www.mgh.harvard.edu/health_info.html*
Mayo Clinic: *www.mayoclinic.com/findinformation/diseasesandconditions/index.cfm*

Books and Brochures

Stripping Away The Barriers To A Healthy Heart: You can Reduce Your Risk of Coronary Heart Disease. Krames Communications, 312 90th Street, Daly City, CA 94015–1898.

Little Book of Heart Wisdom: Living Life To Its Fullest. Cliggott Communications, 55 Holly Hill Lane, P.O. Box 4010, Greenwich, CT 06831–0010.

Cholesterol And Your Heart. American Heart Association, 7272 Greenville Avenue, Dallas, TX 75231–4596.

Cholesterol Control (A Patient's Guide). Health Trend Publishing, P.O. Box 7390, Menlo Park, CA 94026.

You Can Control Your Cholesterol: A Guide to Low-Cholesterol Living. Krames Communications, 312 90th Street, Daly City, CA 94010–1898.

Optimizing Cholesterol Management. Liberty Communications Network, Inc. Windsor Corporate Center, 50 Millstone Rd., East Windsor, NJ 08520.

The Wellness Way Blood Pressure Control. Krames Communications, 1100 Grundy Lane, San Bruno, CA 94066–3030.

Blood Pressure: How To Keep Your Numbers Healthy. International Health Awareness Center, Inc., 350 E. Michigan, Suite 301, Kalamazoo, MI 49007–3851.

Stop High Blood Pressure Before It Stops You. Krames Communications, 1100 Grundy Lane, San Bruno, CA 94066–3030.

Smoking and Heart Disease. American Heart Association, National Center, 7272 Greenville Avenue, Dallas, TX 75231–4596.

Food For Thought: How to Eat for a Healthier, Longer Life. International Health Awareness Center, Inc., 350 E. Michigan, Suite 301, Kalamazoo, MI 49007–3851.

Eating A Heart Healthy Diet. Novartis Pharmaceuticals Corp., East Hanover, NJ 07936.

Aerobic Exercise: The Heart of Your Fitness Program. Krames Communications, 1100 Grundy Lane, San Bruno, CA 94066–3030.

Arrhythmias. Health Trend Publishing, P.O. Box 7390, Menlo Park, CA 94026.

Exercise Thallium Scars. Health Trend Publishing, P.O. Box 7390, Menlo Park, CA 94026.

Cardiac Catheterization. Health Trend Publishing, P.O. Box 7390, Menlo Park, CA 94026.

Electrophysiology (EP) Study. Health Trend Publishing, P.O. Box 7390, Menlo Park, CA 94026.

Understanding Coronary Angioplasty. Krames Communications, 1100 Grundy Lane, San Bruno, CA 94066–3030.

Coronary Stents. Health Trend Publishing, P.O. Box 7390, Menlo Park, CA 94026.

Catheter Ablation. Health Trend Publishing, P.O. Box 7390, Menlo Park, CA 94026.

Understanding Pacemakers. Krames Communications, 1100 Grundy Lane, San Bruno CA 94066–3030.

Implantable Cardioverter Defibrillator (ICD). Health Trend Publishing, P.O. Box 7390, Menlo Park, CA 94026.

After A Heart Attack. Health Trend Publishing, P.O. Box 7390, Menlo Park, CA 94026.

Mayo Clinic Heart Book. William Morrow Publishers, Mayo Clinic, Rochester, MN.

All About Heart Bypass Surgery. Trahair R. Oxford University Press, New York, NY.

Diagnosis: Heart Disease: Answers To Your Questions About Recovery and Lasting Health. Farquhar JW and Spiller GA. W.W. Norton & Co.

Coronary Angioplasty. Clark DA. John Wiley & Sons Publishers, 1991.

Appendix

149

Glossary

Achalasia: Disorder in which the valve in the lower esophagus fails to open properly to allow food to enter the stomach. Instead, food back up into the esophagus, leading to chest pain.

Adrenergic inhibitors: Medications occasionally used to treat hypertension.

Ambulatory (Holter monitor) ECG test: Noninvasive diagnostic test that records the electrical activity of the heart for 24 hours using a portable tape recorder to detect any abnormality of heart rhythm.

Anastomosis: Surgical bypass graft.

Anemia: A decrease in the red blood cells and/or hemoglobin content of the blood.

Angiotensin-converting enzyme (ACE) inhibitors: One of the commonly used heart medications for a variety of cardiac disorders, such as congestive heart failure.

Aneurysm: Bulging and thinning of a blood vessel wall or a heart chamber wall.

Aneurysmectomy: Surgical resection of an aneurysm.

Angina pectoris: Chest pain or chest discomfort caused by insufficient blood supply to the heart muscles as a result of narrowing of the coronary arteries.

Antagonistic effect: Opposing effect.

Anti-anginal drugs: Medications used for the prevention and treatment of angina pectoris (e.g., propranolol or nitroglycerin).

Anti-arrhythmic agents: Medications such as quinidine or procainamide (Pronestyl) used for the prevention and treatment of various cardiac arrhythmias.

Anticoagulants: Medications that interfere with or prevent coagulation of blood (blood clot formation);

common anticoagulants include coumadin and heparin.

Antihypertensive agents: Medications used for the treatment of hypertension.

Aorta: The aorta is the largest trunk-like artery with a diameter about equal to that of a large garden hose. The aorta is connected to the outlet of the left ventricle.

Aortic dissection: Tear of main artery (aorta) leading from the left ventricle.

Aortic valve: The heart valve located at the outlet of the left ventricle.

Arrhythmia: Abnormal heartbeats or rhythm.

Artery: Blood vessel that supplies nutrients and oxygen-rich blood from the heart to various organs and tissues.

Artificial cardiac pacemaker: Electrical device that activates the heart using batteries, used temporarily or implanted permanently; most commonly used in the treatment of various slow heart rhythms, particularly complete AV (heart) block or sick sinus syndrome.

Asthma: Recurrent sudden shortness of breath, with wheezing cough, and sensation of constriction.

Atheroma: Accumulation of fats, cholesterol, and other deposits that often lead to a heart attack.

Atherosclerosis: Hardening of the arteries, the usual cause of angina pectoris and heart attack.

Atria: Plural form of atrium (upper heart chamber).

Atrial fibrillation: Chaotic, irregular, and rapid cardiac rhythm arising from the atria.

Atrial premature contractions: Extra heartbeats arising from the atria.

Atrial septal defect: Hole (abnormal communication) in the muscle wall between the atria, a common form of congenital heart disease.

Atrial septum: A muscular wall between the right and left atria (upper heart chambers).

Atrial tachycardia: Rapid and regular heart rhythm arising from the atria.

Atrium: Receiving (upper) chamber of the heart.

Automatic external defibrillator (AED): Portable defibrillator that can deliver an electrical shock to stop ventricular fibrillation.

AV junctional tachycardia: Rapid and regular heart rhythm arising from the AV junction.

Beriberi heart disease: Cardiomyopathy (heart muscle disease) as a result of vitamin B_1 (thiamine) deficiency.

Beta-blocking agents: Medications such as propranolol (Inderal) commonly used in the treatment of various cardiac arrhythmias, angina pectoris, and hypertension.

Blood pressure (BP): Pressure within the artery—systolic pressure during the pumping phase of the ventricles, diastolic pressure during the expansion period of the ventricles.

Bradyarrhythmia (also bradycardia): Abnormally slow heart rhythm.

Brady-tachyarrhythmia: Combined slow heart rhythm and rapid heart rhythm, often a late sign of the sick sinus syndrome.

Calcium blockers (calcium-channel-blocking agents): Medications to treat high blood pressure, cardiac arrhythmias, and coronary artery disease.

Cardiac arrest: Little or absent heart function as a result of ventricular fibrillation or absent heartbeat.

Cardiac arrhythmia: Abnormal (slow, rapid, or irregular) heart rhythm.

Cardiac catheterization: Invasive diagnostic cardiac test performed by a specially trained cardiologist. Catheters are introduced into the heart chambers and large blood vessels via arm or groin blood vessels. Diagnosis of various heart diseases can be made by measuring pressures in various locations within the heart chambers and blood vessels. This test also identifies the abnormal anatomy of the heart and blood vessels, including the narrowing of coronary arteries.

Cardiac tamponade: Life-threatening heart condition secondary to sudden accumulation of large amounts of fluid or blood in the pericardial sac, leading to marked impairment of the pumping action of the heart.

Cardiogenic shock: Life-threatening complication of a heart attack, common signs of which include hypotension, clammy skin, unclear mental state, markedly reduced urine output, and very poor pumping action of the heart.

Cardiomegaly: Enlarged heart.

Cardiomyopathy: Heart muscle disease.

Cardiopulmonary arrest (collapse): Cessation of heart and lung functions.

Cardiopulmonary resuscitation (CPR): Life-saving technique with two major components (artificial respiration and cardiac massage), used to restore normal functions of the heart and lungs to reestablish delivery of adequate oxygen to vital organs; required immediately for cardiac arrest.

Cardiopulmonary: Heart and lungs.

Cardiovascular system: The entire circulatory system including the heart and the blood vessels.

Cardioverter: Electrical shock machine; defibrillator (DC shock machine).

Catheter ablation (radiofrequency ablation): Nonsurgical treatment (delivery of radiofrequency energy) similar to cardiac catheterization for many kinds of rapid heart rhythms using a specially designed electrode catheter.

Catheter: Small plastic tube.

Cerebral hemorrhage: A form of stroke with hemorrhage (bleeding) in the brain.

Cholecystitis: Inflammation of the gallbladder causing abdominal pain.

Cholesterol: Soft fat-like substance normally present in the body cells, tissues, and blood. However, abnormal levels of cholesterol in the blood are the major coronary risk factors. Normal (desirable) total cholesterol levels are less than 200 mg/dL. There are two kinds of cholesterol LDL (bad) cholesterol and HDL (good) cholesterol.

Cholesterol embolization: Cholesterol clot formation in the bloodstream.

Chordae tendineae: Structures supporting the mitral valve.

Clot busters: Another term for thrombolytic agents.

Collateral circulation: Reserve blood vessels.

Complete AV (heart) block: Disturbance of normal conduction from the atria to the ventricles preventing electrical impulses from traveling through the heart muscle and conduction system, causing a very slow heart rhythm.

Complications: Various medical problems (e.g., heart failure, cardiac arrhythmias) associated with underlying (primary) disease (e.g., heart attack).

Congenital: Arising at birth.

Congestive heart failure: *See* heart failure.

Coronary angiogram (arteriogram): X-ray study in which dye (a chemical) is injected through catheters into the heart chambers and coronary arteries to produce x-ray films that demonstrate the degree and the location of coronary artery narrowing or blockage.

Coronary angioplasty: Dilatation or widening of the narrowed or blocked heart artery using a small plastic tube (catheter).

Coronary artery bypass graft (CABG): Procedure that makes a bypass (detour) to reestablish blood circulation around the blocked segment of the coronary artery, most often using a saphenous vein (obtained from the leg) and less often one or both internal mammary arteries.

Coronary artery: Blood vessel in the heart that supplies nutrients and oxygen-rich blood to the heart muscles.

Coronary artery disease: Heart disease due to narrowing or blockage of coronary arteries from atherosclerosis; commonly used to identify angina pectoris and myocardial infarction.

Coronary risk factors: Various disorders and medical conditions predisposing to a heart attack, commonly including high blood pressure, smoking, and abnormal blood cholesterol levels.

Coronary stent: *See* PTCA.

Cor-pulmonale: Heart disease secondary to lung disease.

Corticosteroids: Cortisone-like medications commonly used in the treatment of various inflammatory processes, such as pericarditis after a heart attack or coronary artery bypass graft.

Costochondritis: Inflammation of the rib cartilage (a fibrous connective tissue).

C-reactive protein (CRP): A specific protein circulating in the blood. Elevated CRP is shown to predispose to a heart attack.

Cyanosis: Purple-blue discoloration of mucous membrane or skin as a result of insufficient supply of blood and oxygen.

Defibrillation: An electric shock applied to the chest to restore the regular heart rhythm.

Diabetes mellitus: Diabetes mellitus is the disorder of sugar metabolism caused by the inability of the body (i.e., pancreas) to produce or respond to insulin properly.

Diastole: Expansion period of the ventricles.

Diastolic murmur: Heart murmur that occurs during the expansion period of the ventricles (pumping chambers).

Digitalis: Inotropic agent that strengthens the pumping action of the heart (better known as heart pill), one of the most important drugs in the treatment of heart failure; commonly used in the treatment of various rapid heart rhythms, particularly atrial fibrillation.

Digitalis intoxication: Digitalis poisoning.

Dilatation: Expansion.

Direct-current shock: Electric shock for rapid heart rhythm.

Diuretic: Water pill that increases the flow of urine.

Dyspnea: Shortness of breath.

Echocardiogram: Noninvasive test using the principle comparable to sonar detection in submarines for the diagnosis and evaluation of various abnormalities in the structures and functions of the heart.

Ectopic beats or rhythms: Heart beats or heart rhythms arising from any location other than the sinus node, originating from the atria, AV junction, or ventricles.

Ectopic focus: Any locations of the heart other than the sinus node.

Edema: Fluid accumulation resulting in swelling, commonly due to heart failure.

Electrocardiogram (ECG or EKG): A recording of the electrical activity of the heart.

Electrolyte imbalance: Abnormal value of one or more electrolytes (e.g., sodium, potassium, chloride, calcium) in the blood.

Electron beam computerized tomography (EBCT): A new special diagnostic test (also known as ultrafast CT scan) to detect calcium within plaques of coronary artery.

Electrophysiologic (EP) study: Insertion of a special electrode catheter into the veins and thence into the heart (similar to cardiac catheterization) to identify the exact site causing life-threatening arrhythmias.

Embolism: Blood clot formation in the blood vessel leading to disturbance of blood circulation to various organs, such as the lungs.

Endocarditis: Bacterial (most commonly staphylococcal and streptococcal) infection of the inner lining of the heart chambers, often affecting damaged heart valves and congenital defects.

Endothelium: The inner layer of a blood vessel.

Esophagitis: Inflammation of the esophagus.

Esophagus: Feeding tube connecting the mouth and stomach.

Event recorder: Form of ambulatory ECG device that records only when an arrhythmia occurs.

Exercise ECG test: Noninvasive diagnostic test for coronary artery disease using a motor-driven treadmill, bicycle, or certain chemicals.

Extrasystoles: Premature heartbeats arising from the atria, AV junction, or ventricles.

Functional capacity: Ability to perform physical activity.

Gland: Certain tissue structure with a specific function of the human body such as the thyroid gland.

Heart block: Slower-than-usual or absent conduction of the cardiac impulse from the atria to the ventricles.

Heart failure: Condition in which the heart is unable to pump blood adequately, causing various symptoms (e.g., shortness of breath, leg edema) and common complication of hypertension and heart attack.

Heart murmur: Abnormal noise generated by blood flow through a damaged heart valve or a congenital defect of the heart. Also called **congestive heart failure**.

Hemodynamic monitoring: Measurement of pressures in various heart chambers and large blood vessels and the determination of oxygen content in blood samples obtained from these chambers and blood vessels.

Hemopericardium: Accumulation of blood in the pericardial sac.

Hemothorax: Accumulation of blood in the chest cavity.

Hiatal hernia: Herniation of a portion of the stomach through the diaphragmatic-esophageal hiatus into the chest, leading to chest pain.

Homocysteine: Form of chemical considered to be a coronary risk factor if found in abnormally high blood levels in the blood.

High-density lipoprotein: A cholesterol that actually protects the arteries against the build-up of fatty deposits, hence the term "good cholesterol" commonly used to designate HDL cholesterol (the desirable level of HDL cholesterol being above 35 mg/dL).

Hyperlipidemia: Elevated levels of cholesterol or triglycerides (or both) in the blood.

Hypertension: Elevated blood pressure, the most common cause of heart failure and the major risk factor for a heart attack.

Hyperthyroidism (thyrotoxicosis): Increased function of the thyroid gland, a common cause of rapid heart rhythms, particularly atrial fibrillation.

Hypotension: Lower-than-normal blood pressure, a common sign of cardiogenic shock.

Hypothyroidism (myxedema): Decreased function of the thyroid gland, a frequent cause of pericarditis and pericardial effusion.

Idiopathic: Arising from an unknown cause.

Implantable cardioverter-defibrillator (ICD): Small electronic device implanted in the chest to deliver an electrical shock automatically when ventricular fibrillation or tachycardia develops.

Inotropic agents: Medications such as digitalis and isoproterenol (Isuprel), used to improve the pumping actions of the heart.

Inferior vena cava: The large vein connected to the right atrium that collects blood from the area of the body below the heart.

Ischemia: Insufficient blood supply to the tissues.

Lipids: Cholesterol and triglycerides.

Lipoproteins: Special carriers that are essential in circulating cholesterol in the blood. The most important lipoproteins are low-density lipoprotein (LDL) and high-density lipoprotein (HDL).

Lithotripsy: Noninvasive treatment to destroy kidney stones.

Long Q-T syndrome: Inherited medical disorder that often produces ventricular fibrillation and sudden death.

Low-density lipoprotein: Often called "bad cholesterol" because elevated LDL is the major coronary risk factor (desirable LDL levels being less than 130 mg/dL).

Magnetic resonance imaging (MRI): A form of special diagnostic x-ray tests for multiple purposes such as detection and precise location and size of a tumor mass in any intestinal organs (e.g., liver cancer). At present, MRI can be used to diagnose coronary artery narrowing or blockage.

METs: Metabolic units or metabolic equivalents, multiple of the basal metabolic unit.

Mitral valve: The valve located between the left atrium (left upper chamber) and left ventricle (left lower chamber).

Mitral valve regurgitation: Leaking back of blood from the left ventricle into the left atrium as a result of a damaged mitral valve.

Myocardial imaging: Nuclear scanning or radioisotope study of the heart, a very useful diagnostic test to detect heart muscle damage or areas of myocardial ischemia.

Myocardial infarction (MI): Heart attack, an event in which a portion of the heart muscle dies as a result of loss of blood supply caused by blockage of one or more coronary arteries.

Myocardial ischemia: Insufficient blood supply to the heart muscle as a result of coronary artery narrowing, leading to angina pectoris.

Myocarditis: Inflammation of the heart muscle.

Myocardium: Heart muscle.

Nuclear scan: Useful diagnostic test to identify blood flow problems to the heart, used to diagnose coronary artery disease.

Occlusion: Blockage.

Omega–3 fatty acids: Substances found to be protective against coronary artery diseases, including heart attack; present in large amounts of oily fish (e.g., salmon and mackerel).

Oxygenated blood: Blood carrying oxygen and nutrients.

Palpitation: Unusual or abnormal feeling in the chest (e.g., feeling of skipped heartbeats, heaviness, or rapid or irregular heartbeating) as a result of various arrhythmias.

Pansystolic (or holosystolic) murmur: Heart murmur that occupies the entire period of the pumping action of the heart.

Papillary muscle: Tissue supporting the mitral valve.

Percutaneous transluminal coronary angioplasty (PTCA): Standard revascularization procedure to open up narrowed or blocked coronary arteries using a specially designed balloon at the tip of a catheter and implantation of a coronary stent (expandable metal mesh tube) is commonly performed to prevent restenosis of the coronary artery.

Pericardial effusion: Fluid accumulation in the pericardial sac.

Pericardial friction rub: Abnormal heart sound (scratching sound) heard by using a stethoscope. It also causes a sensation similar to that of touching a purring cat, an important sign of pericarditis.

Pericardiocentesis (pericardial tap): Aspiration of pericardial fluid via a needle inserted into the pericardium, the best therapeutic approach for massive pericardial effusion or cardiac tamponade.

Pericarditis: Infection or inflammation involving pericardium, commonly due to virus infection but possible after a heart attack or coronary artery bypass graft.

Pericardium: Sac surrounding the heart.

Perioperative myocardial infarction: Myocardial infarction (heart attack) occurring during or immediately after a heart surgery (usually coronary artery bypass graft).

Peripheral pulse: Pulse in the arms or legs (e.g., pulse in the wrist).

Platelet: A kind of blood component that speeds up blood clot formation.

Plaques: *See* Atheroma.

Pleurisy: Inflammation of the membrane that lines the chest cavity and covers the lungs. Pleurisy causes chest pain.

Pneumothorax: Collapse of part or all of a lung as a result of accumulation of air in the chest cavity.

Prinzmetal's angina: Less common type of angina due to the spasm of one or more coronary arteries.

Propranolol (Inderal): Beta-blocking drug effective in treating abnormal heart rhythm, hypertension, and angina pectoris.

Pulmonary edema: Fluid accumulation in the lungs usually due to severe heart failure.

Pulmonary embolism: Blood clots in the lung arteries.

Pulmonary hypertension: Elevated blood pressure in the arteries carrying blood to the lungs.

Pulmonic (pulmonary) valve: The heart valve situated at the outlet of the right ventricle.

Quinidine: Drug that controls and treats abnormal heartbeats and rhythm.

Radiofrequency (RF) ablation: Special electrical treatment to manage a variety of rapid heart rhythms.

Shingles (herpes zoster): Disorder caused by virus (same as that producing chicken pox) that can cause intense pain along the nerve distribution.

Sick sinus syndrome: Dysfunction of sinus node resulting in abnormally slow heart rhythm and leading to dizziness, near-syncope, or syncope.

Sinus node: Natural pacemaker of the heart.

Stenosis: Narrowing.

Stent: *See* Coronary stent and PTCA.

Stress test: Test that evaluates how the heart and blood vessels respond to exertion and may allow diagnosis of coronary artery disease; may be performed using a treadmill or various chemicals (e.g., dobutamine, adenosine).

Superior vena cava: The large vein connected to the right atrium that collects blood from the body area above the heart.

Supraventricular: Any location above the ventricles, namely in the atria or in the A-V node.

Sympathetic system: The sympathetic system is a nerve system that releases "noradrenalin" and speeds up the heart rate.

Syncope: Loss of consciousness as a result of temporary cessation of respiration or circulation, or very slow or rapid heart rhythm.

Synergistic effect: Intensifying effect.

Systole: Contraction (pumping) period of the ventricles.

Systolic murmur: Heart murmur occurring during a pumping period of the ventricles (pumping chambers).

Tachycardia: Rapid heart rhythm. Also called **tachyarrhythmia**.

Thrombolytic therapy: Intravenous administration of medications (e.g., streptokinase, urokinase, tPA, or alteplase) that dissolve blood clots blocking the coronary arteries.

Thromboembolic phenomenon: Blood clot formation.

Thrombophlebitis: Painful and swollen tissues covering inflamed veins, often leading to blood clot formation.

Thrombosis: Blood clot formation within a blood vessel.

Tietze's syndrome: Costochondritis, a condition in which the cartilage of the rib cage, particularly that joining the ribs to the sternum (breastbone), becomes inflamed due to unknown causes and often triggers chest pain.

Tilt table test: Useful diagnostic tool to evaluate fainting spells (syncope or near-syncope).

Tricuspid valve: The heart valve located between the right atrium and the right ventricle.

Triglyceride: Another form of lipid, a lesser coronary risk factor (the desirable triglyceride level being less than 200 mg/dL).

Type A personality: A person with an aggressive, ambitious, and competitive character.

Vagus (or vagal) system: The vagus system is an inhibitory nerve system that tends to slow the heart rate.

Vasculitis: Group of disorders that causes inflammation of the blood vessels.

Vasodilator agents: Medications such as sodium nitroprusside (Nipride) or hydralazine (Apresoline) used in treating severe heart failure and cardiogenic shock.

Vasopressor agents: Medications such as metaraminal (Aramine) or norepinephrine (Levophed) used in treating cardiogenic shock.

Vein: Blood vessel that carries back to the heart oxygen-poor blood and waste products from various organs and tissues.

Ventricle: Pumping chamber of the heart.

Ventricular aneurysm: Thinning and building of the ventricular muscle wall that may lead to ventricular rupture

Ventricular fibrillation: Life-threatening, chaotic, irregular, and ineffective heart rhythm arising from the ventricles, the most common cause of cardiac arrest and frequently a precursor of sudden death.

Ventricular premature contractions: Extra heartbeats arising prematurely from the ventricles.

Ventricular septal defect: Hole (abnormal communication) in the muscle wall between the ventricles, a common form of congenital heart disease and possibly caused by a heart attack; a life-threatening complication.

Ventricular septum: A muscular wall between the right and left ventricles (lower heart chambers).

Ventricular tachycardia (VT): Regular and rapid cardiac rhythm arising from the ventricles, a serious arrhythmia.

Wolff-Parkinson-White syndrome: Form of congenital anomaly (extra electrical pathway between the atria and the ventricles) that often causes various rapid heart rhythms.

Index